Silent Struggler

Silent Struggler

A Caregiver's Personal Story

Dr. Glenn Mollette

Inspiration
Newburgh, Indiana
A Division of GMA Publishing

Edited by Gloria Beanblossom
Cover by Christina Gubbins

Printed in the United States of America

Affectionately dedicated to

Karen, Jared and Zachary

Contents

Introduction

1 Bad News   1
2 A Life of Dedication and Perfection   7
3 MS Rears its Ugly head   13
4 Elected by Acclamation as President of the KBC   21
5 From Walking to a Wheelchair   25
6 Encourage and Allow Independence   35
7 It's Different When It's You   43
8 What Do Caregivers Do?   47
9 Dealing With the Desire to Abandon Ship   55
10 Overcoming the Paranoia of Pushing a Wheelchair   59
11 A Complete Change of Lifestyle   63
12 What Happens to Sex?   69
13 Wild Mood Swings   77
14 Coping With the Suicidal Threats of the Patient   87
15 Coping with Stress   95
16 Exercise   101
17 Be Careful About What You Eat   109
18 You Must Have A Life   115
19 Let Others Help   121
20 What People Expect of You as a Caregiver   129

Table of Contents continued

21 Down They Go and Everybody Else with Them   137
22 What About Guilt   141
23 Trust and Its Impact on Relationships   145
24 Medical Costs   153
25 Housing Becomes a Major Issue   161
26 Traveling with the Patient   165
27 Shopping for my Wife   171
28 You Better Have a Sense of Humor   177
29 Going Out to Eat   181
30 Patience   187
31 Fear   191
32 Trying Everything   195
33 There is Always Somebody Worse   201
34 Who Would Have Thought?   205
35 How Is Karen Doing?   209
36 Try to Understand   215
37 The Dying Process   219
38 For Karen   227
39 From 1998 to November 2000   247

Introduction

Silent Struggler...

I am one of you--one of the "silent strugglers". I wake every morning to see my wife of twenty-four years, the mother of my children, and love of my life, wasting slowly away.

My wife Karen suffers from multiple sclerosis. We received the news that would forever and completely alter our lives in the winter of 1990.

In the last ten years, I have witnessed a woman who seemingly had everything: a loving husband, two healthy sons, a rewarding career; reduced to an invalid, confined to a wheel chair. Karen's battle with MS has left her physically and emotionally scarred, and our family irrevocably changed.

Perhaps, I need to write this book for Glenn Mollette. Perhaps, I need to write this book for Karen. I'm not really sure I have the answer to that question. Friends and family have said, "Oh, that's good therapy for you." Good therapy? Rehashing and rethinking some of the darkest moments of my life--it certainly hasn't been easy or cathartic. It's been painful.

But one thing I am certain of I need to do it for you and all the "silent strugglers" who like myself are traveling down this long treacherous road. I want you to know you aren't alone in all this. I understand. I feel your pain. I know what it is to watch someone you love die little by little, inch by inch.

As a young seminary student, there were no course studies entitled, "caring for a sick wife" or "how to seminars" for pastors whose lives were crumbling all around them. People see me on Sunday morning, standing in the pulpit and think I have a direct line to God. My contact with God is the same as every other believer, and my trials are the same too.

I am no hero. I simply do what I must. I struggle daily with frustration, and most of all exhaustion, and the temptation to wallow in self-pity--to quit--to run.

I initially entitled this book "Silent Struggler -- Journey of a Caregiver," because we are on a long journey. I have no idea how long I must travel this road, and I wish with every fiber of my being that I could end this lonely sojourn, but I cannot.

This book is not a roadmap. It does not offer pat answers or espouse false hope. "Silent Struggler" is my personal account of what it has meant to me to be a caregiver. It is my devout hope that it will give you strength and comfort in your own journey as a silent struggler.

Chapter 1

Bad News

Most people remember the time, place and circumstances surrounding them when bad news comes knocking at the door. I was in the third grade when my teacher announced President John F. Kennedy had been shot. I was pulling into the parking lot of an auto parts store when I heard the news of Elvis' death. I heard about the space shuttle explosion that took the lives of those astronauts, including a schoolteacher, while I was in my office. I was in a motel room with my family in Orlando, Florida where we watched the police cars following a white Ford Bronco and O.J. Simpson. I was in Louisville, Kentucky at Walnut Street Baptist Church when I received the news that my wife Karen had been diagnosed with multiple sclerosis.

Bad news is no respecter of persons. I was thirty-four years old and Karen was thirty-five. I was the newly elected President of the Kentucky Baptist Pastor's Conference. This was a big step up the ladder for me as a pastor and church leader. Being President of the State Pastor's Conference meant I would be in charge of planning the program for the next Pastor's Conference in Paducah, Kentucky, and that I was held in high esteem as "pastor to the pastors", serving over 2200 pastors and churches throughout Kentucky. And it also meant that I was in line for bigger and better things; namely, President of the Kentucky Baptist Convention.

This new position meant my name and picture, along with interviews and press releases, would become commonplace in the state Baptist paper. I had served as a journalist for the "Western Recorder," a weekly Baptist paper for almost ten years, establishing a reputation not only as a journalist, but also as a highly talented and successful pastor. Needless to say, my success at such a young age was heady, the stuff of which egos are fed. And my ego had grown and was growing.

I had just arrived at Walnut Street Baptist Church in Louisville in February of 1990. I had checked into the Hampton Inn where one of my buddies, Bill Messer and I were sharing a room for the state evangelism conference. I had unpacked my clothes, showered and put on one of my best suits to attend the afternoon session of the conference.

People in high positions have friends. If you are a businessperson, an elected official, or are ostensibly wealthy-- you have friends. Or should I say, people who give the appearance of being your friend. Entering the facility I was greeted by friendly smiles, handshakes and congratulatory remarks that accompany a newly elected position.

Observing that the lower level of the church was filled to capacity, I was about to proceed to the balcony, when a voice over the PA system announced, "Glenn Mollette, you have an emergency message and need to call home right away." What on earth could that be? I wondered. Making a quick 180-degree turn, I headed back down the balcony, and made my way to the courtesy desk. I called Karen expecting to hear that perhaps the car had broken down, or one of the kids had fallen out of a tree. Instead I was greeted with the news that was to change all our lives. "Glenn, I have multiple sclerosis."

"What?" I asked, unable to disguise the anxiety in my voice.

"Dr. Wheeler says I have multiple sclerosis."

Karen had noticed some vision change, nothing dramatic, just a change. She made an appointment with Dr. Charles Wheeler, an ophthalmologist in Pikeville, Kentucky. It was in the process of the eye exam that he saw what appeared to be signs of the disease.

In that five-minute conversation, a hundred people surely walked by that desk. Time and space--my whole world came to an abrupt standstill.

Telling Karen I loved her and that I would be home early the next day, I hung up the telephone. I felt very alone and isolated in that throng of people. There were still the congratulatory handshakes, and greetings of, "Glenn you're doing a great job as pastor of your church," but I knew something had just occurred. Those four simple words, "I have multiple sclerosis," would change everything.

Walking back into the main auditorium of the church, I found a seat and sat quietly. My mind was now a million miles away. I was in a state of shock. My body was almost numb. Somebody was up at the podium speaking. I don't know who it was or what they said. I just tried to sit quietly-- all the time wondering if this were a dream or some kind of nightmare.

Back at the hotel that evening, Bill Messer and I would talk. Only nine months earlier Bill had preached a funeral for Karen and I. We had delivered a full term stillborn baby. It was not until the day of delivery that Karen found out from her doctor that there was no heartbeat. The baby was dead. The planned Caesarian birth would have to be done anyway.

I went into the delivery room praying the doctor had made a grave error. But he was right. The baby was dead. It was a full day of sitting and crying for the both of us. For about three hours, I sat and held my beautiful, dead, baby boy--Jesse Caleb. Three days later, Karen and I sat at the graveside, in Paintsville, Kentucky while 150 mourners wept with us over the death of our son.

Losing the baby was devastating for Karen. She lamented month after month the loss of our son, the baby that had once moved so frequently inside her. The emotional trauma was beginning to tell on her physical well being, producing a number of grave physical problems.

Sleep was impossible. I couldn't get Karen off my mind. The news had been heart wrenching. Minutes seemed like hours.

Looking at the hotel clock, it was rapidly approaching 1:00 a.m. I got up and began to pack my clothes. Quietly I closed the hotel room door, leaving Bill sound asleep.

Traffic was practically zero. There had been a weather advisory earlier in the evening predicting freezing rain. The weatherman had been right on target. The roads were razor slick. Driving twenty to thirty miles an hour was risky. This is crazy, I thought to myself, as I proceeded onward, hoping the weather would break and the roads would improve.

5

By the time I pulled into our driveway, I knew Karen would be getting up in thirty minutes to dress for school. She taught at the same building where our two sons attended and they traveled together back and forth. She was already up. Karen heard me walk through the door and flung herself into my arms. Sometimes the only thing you can do is hug somebody. After embracing, I had to ask, "Is Dr. Wheeler really sure about this?"

"He was sure," Karen replied.

Chapter 2

A Life of Dedication and Perfection

Sitting down and wringing our hands was not the best plan of action. Karen proceeded to get dressed for school. The two little guys, Zachary and Jared, not comprehending the earthshaking news their family had received got dressed too. Jared was in elementary school, and Zachary was in childcare.

I was exhausted and proceeded to go to bed. Somehow being at home, with Karen off to her teaching job, seemed to make things feel normal. There's something about being home when trouble is brewing.

I knew if the diagnosis were true that our lives would change. I just didn't know exactly when, or how much. We had to see another doctor. We had to get a second opinion. When you are well and healthy you don't think much about physicians and specialists. I was soon to learn that Karen would need to see a neurologist.

7

After three or four hours of sleep, I was up and showering to go to my office at First Baptist Church. I had been pastor of this growing church since July of 1984. I was blessed that Karen was willing to pick up and move, although not very happily. But Karen made the best of Pikeville. She had received her Master's degree from Georgetown College in Kentucky, and soon landed a part-time teaching position in the Pikeville City School System.

Karen was a great teacher. She threw herself body and soul into her work. Perhaps there were times when she was too dedicated. While working on an endorsement for her teaching certificate, she would often stay up until one or two o'clock in the morning perfecting an assignment, and then exhausted, would get up and face a full day of school.

Majoring in music with an emphasis in piano meant long hours of practice and recitals and perfection. Karen was a perfectionist with a capital P. The house, the kid's clothing, her personal dress, and her work, were all done with the same goal in mind--perfection.

Rarely would a month pass that Karen did not hostess some sort of gathering in our home. There were many hours spent counseling small ladies groups, listening to them, encouraging them, and tending to their emotional wounds. This was also a form of therapy for Karen. The loss of our child had been devastating. These sessions allowed her to vent some of her own feelings of frustration and grief.

I loved our son and felt the loss as deeply as Karen, but by this time, I was weary of the constant rehashing of our tragedy. I felt it was time to move on with our lives. A week after the funeral in June of 1989 we sat in a booth at Dairy Cheer in Pikeville. My very words were, "Let's put the death of this baby behind us. You have a great education and a job you enjoy. I'm pastoring a church I love to pastor. Our financial income is good. Let's move on with life. Let's date again. Let's just be lovers and great companions and move on with life."

Karen listened politely, answering with the resounding notification that we were going to try to have another child. Karen wanted a daughter.

It is impossible in a marriage relationship to go forward by yourself. To go forward and accomplish anything, both partners need to be going in the same direction. It was a tug of war trying to talk to Karen about new goals, dreams, travel and aspirations.

During most of 1989 and 1990, having another baby was the theme of our home. It soon became obvious after repeated attempts and failures that another pregnancy would not occur.

Karen suffered from endometriosis, and painful menstrual cycles. When our other children, Jared and Zachary, had been conceived, a surgical procedure had been performed to help clear the fallopian tubes, expediting conception. Unfortunately, Karen did not opt for this procedure, and the pregnancy never occurred.

The experience of "trying to get pregnant," was nightmarish. We had to have sex on a certain day. And then we had to have sex at a certain time of the day. The thermometer was in constant use. Karen repeatedly checked her temperature to find out exactly when she was ovulating. This meant abstaining from sexual relations until the planned time of conception to insure the full potency of my sperm. The lack of spontaneity and the orchestration of our lovemaking created tension. I was weary of the constant stress and turmoil in our home and Karen's obsession with becoming pregnant.

Karen's insatiable hunger for another child was eating away at her. She was miserable, and that misery spilled over onto the boys and I. Karen had become so bitter and depressed about the loss of the baby and her inability to become pregnant, the slightest irregularities, the smallest difficulties would throw her into a rage. These rages were more than a simple fit of temper. Karen would lose control to the point where I feared she might be on the brink of a seizure. Her face would contort, and she would seemingly lose complete control of her emotions, railing and raving at the children and me. It was during this period of emotional instability that Karen was diagnosed with multiple sclerosis.

Chapter 3

MS Rears Its Ugly head

In the midst of this chaos we tried to maintain some semblance of order in our lives. Karen continued to teach school three days a week. I continued to write sermons and do the work of a pastor.

A slight limp was developing in Karen's right leg. At this point it was only a minor annoyance, but by the first of the year, it became obvious to Karen that something pathological was occurring. If this sounds strange, if you are saying to yourself, "Well, of course something is happening to her body, she has MS," let me say simply that we had never accepted the diagnosis of the ophthalmologist. After all, this couldn't be happening to us, to our family. We were young professionals with two great kids. We had the world by the tail.

By the first of the year it was becoming increasingly obvious that we had to have more medical attention. Karen and I were new at seeking medical care. We were naive about the medical profession. Not all doctors are created equal. One of the physicians we consulted decided to perform a spinal tap in hopes of making a definitive diagnosis. This was a nightmarish experience for Karen. It was the first spinal tap this doctor had ever performed. The procedure was a complete failure. The doctor probed Karen's spinal column numerous times without success. Karen was in agony. I am thankful to report that a close friend and nurse was present during the procedure and suggested calling in an anesthesiologist. This was a blessing. The anesthesiologist was able to draw the spinal fluid with the first injection of the needle. It took a week of recuperating in bed before Karen was able to shake the migraine so commonly associated with spinal taps.

The spinal fluid came back clear! There were no signs of multiple sclerosis. Good news or false hope? We knew there was something wrong, but we hoped and prayed for the best-case scenario. We were encouraged.

The summer of 1991 meant a trip to the Southern Baptist Convention in Atlanta Georgia. This was an annual event. Not only did it allow me to keep abreast of current denominational issues, it was also a great family get away.

We had included the boys on this trip. We planned to take in the workshops and festivities at the convention, and then drive from Atlanta to Kissimmee Florida, spend the night, and then drive on to Orlando and check into the Caribbean Resort.

We made it through the first few days of the convention without a hitch. I was unencumbered by denominational responsibilities, freeing us to walk back and forth to convention activities, eat nice meals, and enjoy each other and life.

Wednesday evening we planned to walk through the convention bookstore. We decided to separate, allowing the boys to check out the children's section, while I browsed the displays and gathered information and literature to take back home. As will sometimes happen in a large crowd, I lost sight of Karen and the boys. I searched for them for almost an hour, when I realized I was missing the convention session. I went to the convention hall thinking that perhaps Karen and the boys might be waiting for me there. I went in and looked around but with several thousand people present there wasn't much chance of finding them. At this point I was becoming a little anxious. At the close of the session, I made my way out of the convention hall and back to our hotel to find Karen and the boys waiting for me. Karen was almost as exasperated as I was. We looked at each other and said simultaneously, "I looked everywhere."

"Glenn something is going on," Karen said. "I almost didn't make it back to the hotel."

"What do you mean?" I asked.

"I just could barely walk the distance. I was so tired. My legs were so heavy. We had to walk so slow to get home."

I put Karen's words out of my mind, and got ready for bed. We had a long drive ahead of us. We arrived at Kissimmee Thursday evening in time for us to take a swim and do some laundry. The evening was calm and restful.

The next morning something was wrong. Karen was miserable and uncomfortable, unable to urinate. "I've had trouble since two in the morning. It has been a rough night." Karen's condition worsened as the morning progressed. "I don't see how I can go to Disney World. I'm feeling horrible."

Sickness never comes at the right time. I didn't feel bad. The boys and I were excited about Disney World. We didn't have time for ailments. I was a little exasperated.

"Karen honey, what do you want to do? Do you want to go to the emergency room?" We debated for about an hour on what to do. We were about fourteen or fifteen hours from home. "Do you want to go home?" I asked. Karen was in real discomfort and driving fifteen hours in a mini-van seemed out of the question. I called the Orlando airport and booked a direct flight to Cincinnati, where Karen's family would pick her up.

Leaving the boys behind was a tough decision for Karen. Within a few miles of the airport Karen began to have a change of heart. "No I'm okay. I can make it. This will wear off. I'm going to stay here."

"Okay," I said, "but we all need to make up our mind because your flight leaves in less than an hour. Just be sure you want to stay here."

A minute later, "No I feel really bad. I'm going."

In the mean time I had two panicky kids. They were cranky and disappointed about the possibility of missing Disney World, and on the verge of tears, already missing Mom. It was not a pleasant drive.

We made it to the passenger drop-off area and I helped Karen in with her bags and check in for the flight. She then boarded the tram that took her to the departure terminal. At this point she was barely able to move. I was more than a little concerned about putting her on that plane alone. She waved to us standing on the shuttle holding onto the center post. It was a sad good-bye. Little Zachary, swiped tears from his cheeks, "I'm going to miss Mom."

Suddenly, I had two little guys alone in Orlando. This was a complete change of plans, a very unwelcome change. I had some decisions to make. Did we head directly home? Did we spend the night and then head back, or did we stay and go to Disney World as planned. The boys and I decided to go on to Disney World. It was a very tough decision and there have been times when I have felt very guilty.

All caregivers at one time or another are faced with this kind of decision. It may not be as big or eventful but you will have to make the decision to go on with life, which often means excluding the patient. This is tough. You feel guilty. You are out experiencing the world, while the patient is stuck in a bed or a wheel chair. Plus, you can expect those you know to criticize you. Family and friends and associates will expect more from you, than they would themselves. It has become a constant source of paranoia for me trying to second-guess how people will react. There comes a point in time when you must put that behind you, and simply go on, in the knowledge that you can only do your best, and no more.

By the time Karen made it to Dayton, she was unable to walk. In hindsight, we have come to the conclusion that she was having a multiple sclerosis attack.

Multiple sclerosis attacks strike the victim, much like ocean waves hitting a beach. The disease attacks the nervous system, does a certain amount of damage and then recedes for a period of time. Later, and who knows when or how much later, the patient will suffer another attack. Each episode leaves the patient more debilitated. The patient may eventually lose the use of their arms and legs. Speech becomes slurred and swallowing is difficult. The muscles of the diaphragm begin to weaken and atrophy, causing extreme stress for the lungs, making the simple act of taking a breath an exhausting procedure. Multiple sclerosis is a slow, cruel killer.

Chapter 4

Elected by Acclamation as President of the KBC

It was the middle of summer, the kids were out of school, and my thoughts turned to summer time outings, hot weather, and the Kentucky Baptist Convention. The annual meeting would be in Lexington, Kentucky. This would be the year I would run for President.

As we approached the November convention some issues had to be resolved. If I were elected President I would be the youngest man in the history of Kentucky Baptists to be elected to this position. No one had ever been elected at the age of thirty-six. There was some concern, and frankly a bit of jealously among my colleagues. All to often I would hear, "Maybe Glenn you should wait. You have plenty of time." This would have been true, if my circumstances had been different. But my wife has multiple sclerosis. I knew what was coming for my life and family. I knew I had about two years or perhaps less, to be active in the denomination, before Karen's illness would begin dictating the terms of our lives. I consider myself fortunate, in that I had observed the ravages of multiple sclerosis as a teenager. My pastor's wife died from the horrible disease. This gave me more of an insight into the disease process, and allowed me to make some plans for the future. Not all caregivers are allowed this special dispensation of grace. They find themselves locked into a situation they never could have imagined.

At the Tuesday afternoon session of the convention, I was elected by acclamation to serve as President of the Kentucky Baptist Convention. No one even ran against me. I was stunned. What I had been hoping and praying for had come to pass. I was elated.

I called Karen after the session to give her my wonderful news. She rejoiced with me. Sadly this would not always be the case in the days to come. I think it has to be hard to rejoice with people who are moving on with life. It is a severe test of our character to be happy for others' success when we feel like failures ourselves. Karen would voice this resentment later when she was no longer able to teach school, and was forced to spend more and more time at home. I can't blame her. I would probably be worse, especially if I could not physically get up and do something about it.

The person with multiple sclerosis, muscular dystrophy, terminal cancer or whatever they may be battling, feels the hopelessness of their situation. Their biggest goal for the day may be simply making it to the bathroom without falling. Please understand that this is not true of all MS sufferers, many of whom have goals and aspirations for their lives.

The congregation at First Baptist Church was very nice to me the next Sunday. When I came out for the morning worship service the 600 or so people who were gathered there, stood and gave me a standing ovation for my election as President of the state convention. It was a great feeling of support. Articles from the state Baptist paper and stories in the Lexington Herald appeared over the same weekend. This is just what I needed. My ego was soaring.

Looking back, I wish I had taken it with a grain of salt. Today after spending years with a sick wife and almost living out of sight denominationally, I know I would approach accolades with a more humble spirit. We live and we learn.

The next twelve months would be one of the most difficult years of my life. It would be an education; and unfortunately, sometimes we have to learn our lessons the hard way.

I would be spending far too much time away from home and my church, attending to convention activities in Louisville. One lesson every caregiver must learn is you are limited to how many outside projects you can participate in. I had my plate full.

Chapter 5

From Walking to a Wheelchair

Multiple sclerosis can strike with alarming rapidity, but it can also lay dormant for months, even years. In Karen's case, she was able to continue teaching, playing the piano, and caring for the children three years after the initial diagnosis.

I will always be grateful for those years. But I allowed myself a very costly luxury. I allowed myself to believe that Karen could just snap out of it, the way she snapped in and out of her tantrums and mood swings.

That delusion was shattered in the summer of 1991. Karen, her father and I, went to Mayo Clinic in Rochester, New York. She was subjected to a battery of exhaustive tests. The verdict from the neurology clinic confirmed what I had feared. Karen did indeed, have multiple sclerosis. There was no longer any doubt. She walked down the hospital corridor after spending three hours in the neurology clinic and said, "They say I have MS but that I should be okay. They don't think it's chronic progressive."

"Are they sure? What about the Epstein Barr?" After the episode in Florida, and the emergency plane trip back to Cincinnati, the attending physician who examined her had told Karen, that she had Epstein Barr, or chronic fatigue syndrome.

Karen replied, with guarded optimism, "They don't think I'm going to be any worse and shouldn't have any trouble."

My heart sank. This was definitely not the news I had wanted to hear.

In the days that followed, Karen was often angry, depressed and difficult to understand and live with. I did my best to support and reassure her, but living with a disease like MS isn't easy. It's ever present, even on good days. There is always a sense of uneasiness floating in and out of the unconscious mind. Will it strike again? When will I have another attack? What's to become of me? That sort of pressure, on a daily basis, takes its toll.

Much to Karen's credit, those on the outside looking in, would never have suspected she was ill. Karen continued her daily routine of work, family and church. Every Sunday she would hobble up two flights of stairs to teach a Ladies' Sunday school Class. I'm proud to say her class grew to be the largest in the church.

In the early part of 1992 we held revival services at our church. As was the custom, Karen was the pianist for the services. Karen would sit on the front pew in order to have quick and easy access to the grand piano. When the minister began what we call in Baptist circles, "the hymn of invitation," Karen should have been able to move to the piano in a matter of seconds, but on this occasion she simply could not. It was as if her body was "shutting down." I watched in horror and disbelief as Karen slowly and laboriously limped her way to the piano. This went on Sunday through Wednesday night. At the time, I didn't fully comprehend what was happening to Karen. It is obvious to me now that she was experiencing a multiple sclerosis attack. So often in life we don't know or understand until it's too late.

After this episode, Karen's neurologist from Lexington ordered adrenocorticotrophic hormone (ACTH), a type of steroid or protein type hormone. ACTH was administered to Karen intravenously for five days. After receiving the medication Karen was able to reclaim much of her lost strength and agility. These results usually lasted from three to four weeks after the administration of the drug. Sadly, as time and the disease progressed, the benefits of ACTH began to wane. Soon the effects of the drug lasted only a couple of weeks, then a week, then a day, and then not at all.

There is no one, common rule that applies to the multiple sclerosis patient. In Karen's case, it seems the damage caused by the onset of an attack is irreversible. There simply isn't enough time for the body to recuperate and heal itself fully before the ravages of the disease are again weakening and damaging the patient's nervous system. With the onset of each new attack, more damage is done, leaving the patient more and more debilitated.

During the winter of 1993 it was becoming increasingly difficult for Karen to drive. You can't drive a car if your legs don't work. The next move was to install a handicap hand control system. This system attaches to the brake and gas pedals making it possible to operate them with one single hand control. This device gave Karen a renewed sense of freedom. Once again she could run simple errands or chauffeur the kids to their extra-curricular activities.

In the spring of 1994, we moved to Newburgh, Indiana. I became the pastor of Gateway Baptist Church, and officially began my ministry with the church, January 1, 1994. I was excited about my new pastorate in Newburgh. I saw the possibilities of the community and the church. I felt under the right conditions the church could prosper and do very well.

The Sunday I preached my first sermon at Gateway, Karen was still standing. She could still walk, but she needed to hold onto something. Whenever we entered the sanctuary, Karen had to be holding onto my arm to keep her balance. By the end of April Karen was clinging desperately onto objects and people to bear some of her weight. I knew this situation couldn't continue, and it was then that her father presented her with a walker. This was an emotional issue for me. I knew intellectually that Karen needed the walker, but in my heart I felt we were crossing a line, a line of no return.

The walker may have been upsetting to me, but for Karen it was a real boon. It gave here a sense of mobility and flexibility. No longer did she have to reach for something to balance herself against. Nor did she have to wait for somebody to give her an arm to lean on--she had a walker.

Several months preceding our move to Newburgh we had been in dialogue with Berlex Pharmaceutical Company about a new drug called Beta Interferon or Betaseron. The published studies on Beta Interferon were very encouraging. Beta Interferon was supposed to help the non-chronic progressive MS patient. The concept behind the drug is simple. It was suppose to stop the progression of MS, allowing the nervous system the time needed to repair itself.

We had tremendously high hopes for Beta Interferon. Karen had been taking Copaxon, with no success. We were positive this new drug therapy would be the answer to our prayers. We contacted our neurologist at the Lexington Clinic about the drug.

We learned in early January of 1994 that the Food and Drug Administration had finally released Beta Interferon. The bad news was--availability and cost.

Getting Beta Interferon would not be easy. Four hundred thousand people in the United States have MS. Karen was one among many, clamoring for this miracle in a bottle. Berlex could not accommodate all the requests and therefore dispensed Beta Interferon on a lottery system. Patients were assigned months and years, according to the whim of this lottery, when they could expect to start receiving the drug. In Karen's case, we would be able to get the drug in October. Some people in the lottery had dates set as far in advance as one year. I suppose we should have felt ourselves fortunate, but Karen's condition steadily worsened with each passing day. We were in constant dialogue with our neurologist in Lexington and Berlex, hoping as the old saying goes "the squeaky wheel, gets the grease." Unfortunately, no matter how much we "squeaked," we were told that we were on the list and we would receive the drug as soon as it became available and not before.

We received word from Berlex that we would receive the Beta Interferon in May, almost five months earlier than promised. Surely we believed God had answered our prayers. Surely God was working on our behalf.

In hindsight, I think the pharmaceutical company was able to distribute the drug faster than they had previously thought, and sadly to say, many people just didn't qualify financially. That's right, before we could receive the drug we had to present proof of our ability to pay--a hard cruel fact in our so-called modern society. There must have been thousands on that sterile lottery list that simply could not afford the one thousand-dollar per month expenditure. I'm really rather surprised we were not turned away too. My financial statement was not very impressive.

We selected Wal-Greens of Evansville as the pharmacy where we would in the future be obtaining the Beta Interferon. The day Wal-Greens called with the news that the drug was in, and waiting for us, was more than exciting, we were elated. We felt like we were buying a miracle! We knew this was the very thing that would stop Karen's downward progression.

We waited on pins and needles for our miracle. Two days after the first injection I quizzed Karen, hoping for good news. But it was too early to tell.

Karen stayed on Beta Interferon for almost three years. This was far too long. During this time her condition continued to worsen. And as bad as her physical symptoms were becoming, her emotional health was even more precarious. The drug company failed to tell us the side effects we might expect from the drug. Karen had already suffered from massive bouts of depression. The disease contributes to depression. Add to that a drug with the depressing properties of Beta Interferon, and you have a suicidal situation brewing. I will elaborate more on this in subsequent chapters.

We were determined not to give up. We had heard good reports on a drug called Avonex. It too, was supposed to stop the downward spiral of multiple sclerosis. We tried Avonex for about one year with no results. It was heartbreaking to watch Karen day by day lose more of her physical abilities.

In October of 1994 we bought our first wheelchair. Such a simple, uncomplicated sentence, for what was one of the most heartrending experiences of my life. This was a purchase I dreaded. It was the final and absolute admission that Karen was an invalid. The dye was cast. There was no turning back. We could no longer live in the murky realm of denial; no more false hope.

Reality seems to come in stages. First you hope and pray that the doctor made some dreadful mistake and that soon all will be rectified and life will return to normal. When it becomes all too evident that no mistake was made, anger prevails: anger towards the illness, anger with the doctors, and most of all anger--a burning, aching rage directed at God. "Why God does this have to happen to us? Why me?"

Chapter 6

Encourage and Allow Independence

Through the years since Karen was diagnosed, I have to the best of my ability tried to allow her as much freedom as possible to maintain an active lifestyle. It is painful to watch Karen expending so much time and so much of her limited energy to tasks that she could have accomplished in a matter minutes before the onset of her disease.

I gave a great deal of thought to hiring a housekeeper to come in a few days a week, in the hope of relieving some of Karen's workload. However, upon reflection, I think at this stage the worst thing I could do, would be to say to Karen, "I am going to bring somebody into the house that will do everything you're doing now. She'll wash our clothes, make the beds, run the vacuum cleaner and do the dishes. You won't have to do a thing."

That would be a mistake. Household chores are meaningful tasks to Karen. They give her a sense of fulfillment and completeness. She feels like she is making a contribution to the family. Her efforts at keeping house also give her something to do with her time. It is wonderful for her and our family that she enjoys and feels a need to be busy.

Tinkering around the house gives her a way to channel her energy and keeps her mental outlook healthy.

The house is a passion for Karen. We have had our moments and misunderstandings when I've failed to put the toothpaste away in the morning or left my clothes lying on a chair in the bedroom. My desk and office at times looks as though it's been ravished by a tornado. I get busy and preoccupied with several projects. I channel my energy into the projects at hand. When my project is completed, I make the bed. When my writing or sermon preparation is finished then I worry about straightening my desk.

Karen is just the opposite. There is no peace within her if there is an unmade bed in the house. She could never go to bed with one dirty dish in the kitchen sink. Her obsession with cleanliness and an orderly house has been a source of stress between us. I think it is most regrettable that something as trivial as an unmade bed could cause a falling out between a married couple.

Karen is still determined to be a model housekeeper. The problem is, she is so limited in what she can do. I see her struggle to wheel her chair up to the kitchen sink to wash dishes. I watch her wheel herself around a bed as she carefully makes it to her satisfaction. We have three vacuum cleaners, a normal upright, a hand held vacuum, and a mop vacuum cleaner. Karen bends over the side of her chair to run the hand held vacuum over the tile on the kitchen floor. There are many mornings when I have walked in to find her vacuuming around the house in her wheelchair. It is amazing.

Karen still wants to do the laundry. Currently the boys or I load the washing machine and empty it for her. I have mistakenly put some articles in the dryer I shouldn't have and shrunk them. No wonder Karen is a little mistrusting of my laundry skills. She meticulously sorts through the laundry placing some articles in the dryer while hanging some to dry. It is painful to watch the amount of energy Karen has to expend to accomplish this once simple task.

Of all the household duties Karen still wants to perform, cooking is the biggest ordeal. Cooking requires the ability to move around. You must be able to open the oven door, you have to be able to stoop and reach, open cabinet doors and remove pots and pans.

The boys and I will periodically assist Karen in putting together a simple meal. It is an exhausting and frustrating experience for Karen. Often times in her attempts at perfection she becomes so frustrated she bursts into tears and says things to the boys and I that she will later regret.

At the time of this writing, Karen is still able to drive our van with the aide of hand controls. The hand controls are mounted on the steering column and allow the driver to accelerate or stop the vehicle with the left hand.

When I am not home my eldest son is strong enough to lift his mother into the van and then secure the wheelchair in the rear compartment. When they arrive at the mall or grocery store, he must assemble the wheelchair and then lift Karen from the van and place her in it.

Karen has declined to such a stage that she has to be lifted into the van and placed behind the wheel. She has periodically complained of her arms and hands feeling numb. The day will come when Karen will not have enough strength in her hands to use the hand controls.

This brings me to the question of how far do I go? How long do I continue to allow her to drive? Should I intervene and stop her from driving? Is she a danger to herself? My kids ride with her. Is it really safe for them to be in the car with her behind the wheel?

My stance has been to let her drive as long as she can. It is probably her last true freedom. Driving is something that Karen has always loved to do. In the days before she was diagnosed with MS she would pack up the boys and make the five-hour drive to visit her family in Ohio. Today she drives five miles to go to the grocery store.

The day will come when Karen will not be able to manage the hand controls if the disease continues its current progression. This will be a hard and difficult day for Karen.

When do you say no more driving? This becomes a major issue to children of the elderly. A friend of mine has a mother in her eighties. She is currently living with her son. When it came time to renew her license, the son confided to me, "I hope they won't renew mother's license."

There has to be a mutual understanding between child and parent or caregiver and care receiver that can tolerate suggestions and advice. I want to reiterate, I think Karen should be allowed to drive as long as possible. I think it is mentally and emotionally healthy. But the time will come when I will have to say, "Karen, I think we need a doctor's opinion about this." "Passing the buck," as it were, relieves some of the pressure and resentment that may come your way from a very disappointed and unhappy patient. The loved one who feels that the privilege of driving has not been arbitrarily ripped away from them will be easier to live with and care for.

My birthday is January tenth. Karen and I went to one of our favorite places for dinner to celebrate. When the waitress brought the check Karen wanted to pay for my birthday dinner. I wouldn't let her do it. I guess it is the male ego syndrome. I regret that now. It was something she really wanted to do and I think would have given her pleasure.

Karen receives a small social security disability check each month. It isn't a great deal of money, but it gives her the satisfaction of knowing that she can still contribute monetarily to the family. I felt her money would be better spent on medication or doctor bills rather than for my birthday dinner. This is an area where many caregivers need to learn to bend and allow the loved one to do what they can for them. The patient already feels like a burden upon the family. Bearing the price of a meal or a family outing is a lift to their pride and ego.

The contribution that Karen has continued to make as a parent, can never be replaced. No one can take the place of a caring mother. There were times during her illness when I questioned the effects Karen's emotions had upon the children. There were many difficult days when the kids had to cope with a mother who was unreasonably emotional due to her illness.

In spite of that it has been inspiring to see Karen's commitment to her children and their education. When Zachary was in the second grade he struggled terribly with reading. He was at a total loss. It was the patient steadfast love of his mother who sat with him each night and worked ceaselessly on his reading skills that made the difference for him.

When Zachary was having problems with math Karen was there for him again. In the evenings when I knew she had little strength to give, Karen would wheel up to the kitchen table and do homework with Zachary. Her commitment to help her son in math for hours is a tribute to a mother's heart.

In recent days Karen has been committed to reading to the boys and having prayer with them each night before they go to bed. I have been one to hurry through these devotional times. But Karen being the meticulous person she is never rushes through this most important ritual. When my boys grow up and if they are men of prayer, it will be because of the commitment of their mother.

Encouraging Karen to interact as much as possible with the boys is allowing her to fulfill what is closest to her heart. Her children, her home and feeling a sense of usefulness have been her life.

This is a difficult part of our journey. Watching as those we love struggle to perform tasks that we ourselves take for granted. Love them; encourage them to stay as mobile and independent for a long as possible. You will discover your care and encouragement will ensure a healthier and more productive relationship between caregiver and care receiver.

Chapter 7

It's Different When It's You

I've been in the ministry thirty years. I have officiated at hundreds of funerals. I have stood by bedsides of dying people and consoled them while offering advice and support for the loved ones gathered around the bed watching them die.

I would often have a prayer with the person who was in charge of caring for the sick. I would share a verse of scripture, and extol them to be brave and put their faith in the Lord. Looking back I now realize I didn't have the foggiest notion of what I was doing. I could only imagine what they were going through. As ministers what we tell people they ought to do becomes more personal when suddenly the shoe is on the other foot.

Experiencing the every day drudgery of caring for a chronically ill person is far different and far removed from reading about it. I have a doctorate in "Pastoral Care." Simply stated, this means I have spent years studying how to aid and counsel those who are dealing with life traumas: divorce, grief and emotional problems. I have read books and case studies about suffering and loss. I have even been asked to summarize how I might react to certain situations. I have witnessed first hand the loss of personal dignity and the suffering of those in nursing homes and hospitals. But for all my years of study and eyewitness accounts of suffering, I was completely unprepared to face the trials of a daily caregiver.

There are many well-meaning people who are never weary, it seems, of offering a number of well-worn clichés: "God helps those who help themselves," "Keep your chin up," "Every cloud has a silver lining," and on and on it goes. Or as it often happens, an acquaintance will try to speculate how or what I should be doing as a caregiver. And I must admit, I can recall myself years ago doing exactly the same thing. Other ministers will try to relate to my situation in an attempt to lend a sympathetic ear. Generally, I don't say anything, but I have had a very strong urge on certain occasions to say simply, "Buddy, leave it alone. You don't have a clue."

I know those of you reading this book that find yourselves in my position, can identify with some, if not all of these sentiments.

We belong to a very unique, private club, and the membership dues are high, very high. To belong to this club you must first face the devastating fact that someone you love is ill; terribly, irretrievably ill. Ah but wait, there is more. You have to experience: anger, frustration, grief, complete and literal exhaustion, and the emotional emptiness that comes from knowing that there is really nothing you can do to alleviate this painful situation for yourself or the one you are caring for.

I have had the honor to know some very distinguished members of this club. I could list them here one by one, but that would serve no purpose, for they know who they are, and more importantly the Good Father knows who they are.

I viewed their labor and sacrifice simply as a part of their lives, something they did. It was expected, after all. I bow my head in shame to admit that. I believe I would have taken more notice of their predicament if they would have thrown up their hands in despair and tossed their loved ones out into the street. Yes, then I would have thought, "What a low life. That's terrible of them to treat their loved one that way." Never judge a man until you've walked a mile in his shoes, and to paraphrase, never judge a caregiver until you've walked a mile in his shoes.

I don't pretend to be privy to the thoughts and feelings of everyone who is faced with caring for a chronically ill patient, but I have my suspicions that many are good actors. I know I personally wear many masks. Friends and acquaintances will come up to me and say, "Glenn you are always smiling. Glenn you never complain. Glenn you are always encouraging others." Those are true statements. For one, when you are helping others it seems to take your mind off your own problems. Secondly, nobody wants to hear about my problems. Third, if you are honest and say, "My wife is sick; I'm sick and tired of her being sick. I hate the disease. I am worn out with having to give her a bath and dressing her and lugging her around." If you express those sentiments to anyone other than a very close and caring friend, you will receive some very strange looks. So up goes the mask, and the standard answer issues from your lips, "She's fine, thanks."

You don't know what it feels like to swim until you swim. You can't explain flying until you've flown. You can't explain being in love until you've been in love. And you can't fully explain being a caregiver of the chronically ill until you have to do it--day after day.

Chapter 8

What Do Caregivers Do?

Caregivers cook, clean, do laundry, bathe, dress and feed the patient and serve as an emotional dumping ground for any and all emotional breakdowns. Does that rather long, overwhelming sentence give you pause? It should, because that is the daily duty roster of a caregiver.

On a typical day, I rise before 5:00 a.m. for a much needed run. Exercise and plenty of it, are a mainstay for me. Then it's a quick cup of coffee and time to wake the boys for school. Karen at this point is usually resting on the sofa.

Breakfast for Jared and Zachary is a simple affair, cereal, toast and juice. As soon as the boys are out the door and on the bus my attention turns to Karen.

I lift Karen from the sofa into her wheelchair. I do this by placing my hands under her armpits and as gently as possible pick her up and place her in the chair. I wheel Karen into the bathroom and station her chair beside the bathtub. I remove her socks; people who are afflicted with chronic progressive MS often are unable to wear shoes. I then undress her from the waist down. This means Karen must muster what little strength she has left in her arms and hands to elevate her torso a few inches above the wheelchair seat. This allows me to slide her slacks down over her hips.

Once Karen is undressed, I lift her from the wheelchair and place her on the bath bench. A bath bench is an aid enabling handicapped persons the needed stability to bathe in a conventional bathtub. I'm 6'3 and in good health, however, even though Karen only weighs 120 pounds, she is very difficult to lift and move. The more limited the patient becomes in their capacity to function the more difficult the task of lifting, moving and repositioning becomes.

The bath bench does not allow Karen to be submerged in the water. In order to bathe we turn the faucet on and let the water run throughout the bath. With a washcloth and soft soap Karen is still able at the time of this writing to bathe and wash her hair. There are days when it is more difficult for her than others, but it is important for Karen to be as independent as possible. The more the boys and I do for her, the less independent she becomes.

After the bath has been completed, I help Karen back into her wheelchair, first ensuring that one of three pillows is situated correctly on the seat.

Unfortunately one of the problems associated with MS is lack of bladder control. The pillows make it much easier for

Karen to transfer from her wheelchair to the handicap toilet seat.

A pillow also offers more flexibility and comfort for Karen. Karen suffers tremendously from pressure sores. At the present time we have been nursing a pressure sore on her hip the size of a golf ball. It is angry, red and inflamed, bleeding at the least provocation, hence the need for the pillows and painkillers. Without them Karen would lose her mind from the constant, nagging pain.

Dressing Karen starts from the waist down, much the way you would dress a baby. This means putting on a bladder pad and underwear. Once the bladder pad and underwear is positioned, she uses her hands and arms to elevate her torso so I can slip them up and over her hips. Her slacks or skirt is managed in much the same fashion, and then her stockings. Karen also requires some help with her blouse. Basically this means helping her with one arm at a time, just like a gentleman would help a lady with her coat.

Breakfast is next on the agenda. Again, it is usually simple fair: cereal, fruit, toast and juice. Cooking is not my forte. One difficulty Karen and I have had to deal with is, we simply do not get along in the kitchen. Her ideas and mine about cooking are quite different. She has generally been good about eating whatever I can throw together. Sadly, Karen has reached the point where food is secondary to a host of other concerns. Namely, "How will I get off the couch and into my wheelchair. Will I be able to slide off my wheelchair onto the toilet seat?" When a person is faced with these daunting questions, food preparation slides to the bottom of the priority list.

Now I must shower, shave and prepare for my day as the pastor of a growing, active church. Karen has a portable telephone near her in case the unforeseen should happen. Sadly, on more than one occasion I have received calls at my office from Karen, crying and distraught because she'd fallen from her wheelchair and was unable to get up. That's part of my day too. As a caregiver, you're always on call. No matter what else you may be doing, there is the ever- present concern at the back of your mind about the patient. Have they fallen? Do they need me? The mental weight can be mind numbing.

I come home to fix lunch, and much to my embarrassment, I have to admit, I often stop for fast food. As I mentioned, cooking is not my forte. After lunch Karen usually rests on the couch until dinner. After dinner she is in her chair doing what she can do. Karen is very particular about her home, and still enjoys overseeing the laundry and folding clothes. She also spends a good portion of her evening talking to the boys and helping with homework assignments.

At bedtime, Karen requires another bath and her medications. I am usually exhausted and keeping a good attitude can become quite difficult, especially if Karen has had a difficult day and is feeling depressed and negative.

Imagine if you will anything else that has to been done around the house, it's the caregiver's responsibility to handle it. From the smallest to the largest problems, it's all on the caregiver's shoulders. The daily grind is endless.

Karen, like the rest of us enjoys an outing. This is another task assigned to the caregiver.

In order to seat Karen in the car I must position her wheelchair at just the right angle to the passenger door. I then lift her up and place her lower back against the seat. At this point I brace my knee against her thighs to steady myself and keep her from falling. I then proceed to lift her left leg and slide it into the car. Lifting her right leg, I then slide her as gently as I can into the seat. I have never dropped Karen during this procedure, but there have been a few times when I almost fell. I have tripped on the wheelchair and have gotten twisted and off balance lifting her into position. I then collapse the wheelchair and place it in the back of the car. This entire process must be repeated on the return trip home.

I have to say, I am grateful to have a garage. It affords us a sense of privacy. It is impossible to lift an invalid into a car smoothly. At best a shoe will come off in the process or Karen's slacks or skirt will become disarranged. This is very irritating to someone like Karen, who has always been so fastidious about her personal appearance. The garage allows us a few minutes for Karen to vent her frustrations and make the necessary adjustments to her clothing.

Before bringing this chapter to a close, I want to add that I am not the only caregiver in our home. Our children travel the same road we do. Every move we make and every decision affects them.

In a home where there is a chronically ill parent, the children become a part of the care giving cycle. It is inescapable. There is no denying the reality of the situation the child finds himself in. When one muscle in the body hurts the whole body hurts. When one family member hurts everybody else hurts.

Children aren't born into this world to nurture an ailing parent. They are conceived and presented to us as a most precious gift to be validated and loved. Their world consists of schoolmates, football games, rock stars and dreaming of the future.

My sons have had to make many sacrifices along the way, but I am proud to say, with very little complaint. The boys and I have had to forego a tremendous amount of father son time; just the guys, fishing and camping trips, because we just couldn't leave mom at home. I think that is one of my deepest regrets. But through it all, the boys, Jared and Zachary have been wonderful. A father couldn't ask for two finer sons.

Chapter 9

Dealing With the Desire to Abandon Ship

We are sustained and strengthened by different motivating factors. We go to work, we marry, have children, divorce, stay with a marriage, go to church, quit church, exercise, eat too much and on and on. We are motivated by what we think we need, the expectations of the world, and what we think will make us happy and fulfilled.

Living day in and day out with a chronically ill person who is totally dependent on you for their very survival is not a very pleasant prospect. There is nothing motivating about bedpans, soiled undergarments and bouts of hysteria and depression. This person is no longer the loving companion of your youth, or the kind understanding parent. Illness brings change. And it is not a positive change.

The caregiver, whether they are the spouse, parent or child, begs the question: How much longer--how much longer can I do this?

I know I have personally wrestled with this dilemma. True, I've been with Karen for the 24 years of our marriage. I've been "Johnny on the spot" since we received the diagnosis in 1990. But still every day I ask myself the question, "Can I continue to do this? How long Lord, can I last?" Can I continue to remain at her side for another twenty or more years? Do I have the stamina to bathe my wife, dress her, and be within a few minutes of the house to pick her up off the floor if she falls?

These are tough questions. No that's an understatement. They are hard, excruciating questions to deal with on a day-to-day basis.

To compound the guilt and feelings of inadequacy, friends and acquaintances come up and pat me on the back, and marvel, "Glenn I don't know how you do it?" If I voiced my true feelings, if I cried out in despair that I was discouraged and tired, and that I feel like walking out and quitting--what would their response be? Would they be understanding and sympathetic, or would they be thinking, "What a louse that guy is."

So, as a caregiver and one of the silent strugglers, I keep my feelings locked within, and plant one foot in front of the other. We stay quietly and tediously without any fanfare, recognition or reward. At least the rewards may not seem to be there. But they are dear friends. We don't receive all our rewards in this life. There is a greater reward yet to come.

I have thought to myself on sleepless nights, when all I had to sustain me were adrenaline and raw nervous energy,

"It can't get any worse than this, it just can't." But it can, and it has. There have been days when I just wanted to run, to abandon ship, as it were. But would that make me happy? What of my children, whom I love more than my own life? Who would be there for them, if I were gone? Would Karen spend her final days languishing in a nursing home or long term care facility, surrounded by strangers?

I know my in-laws love Karen very much and will do what they can to help her. They are good people. But they don't want Karen at home to care for over the long haul. A brief visit for a few days is all right. It would be a nightmarish experience for them to have her in their home on a permanent basis. There have been times when Karen has had severe emotional problems and outbursts of rage. "We don't want her coming back here and upsetting our home," has been the stern resounding comment that I have heard from her mother and sister. Once again I must carry the burden.

We are told that we are never given a burden to heavy to bear. I believe this with all my heart. At one time or another every one of us will have some kind of cross to bear. Jesus carried his. And we can carry ours without pouting and sulking. We can live life with a bounce in our step and a smile on our face. We can be more than conquerors through Christ who loves and cares for us. In His Word He told us to remain in Him. "I am the vine; you are the branches. If a man remains in me and I in him, he will bear much fruit; apart from me you can do nothing" (John 15:5). "If a man remains in me and my words remain in you, ask whatever you wish, and it will be given you" (John 15:7). Does that mean that all are problems will be taken from us simply by asking? Will the Good Father restore Karen to the woman she was before MS entered our lives? Only He can know these things, but of one thing I am absolutely certain, you can overcome and be victorious in your life through His grace and abiding love. The Lord is our shepherd. We need not fear. He will be with us unto the end. So fear not dear friends and do not be discouraged.

I have made the personal commitment to stay with Karen. I'm not mad about it nor do I want sympathy or applause. I vowed to Karen on our wedding day to be faithful to her in sickness and in health. I hold those vows sacred. I stay from a sense of responsibility to her and our children, but most importantly I stay because of love. Karen is crippled and in a wheelchair, but she is still amazingly beautiful. I deeply love her. Love has a way of enabling you to go the second mile. Love sees us through. There is power in love.

Chapter 10

Overcoming the Paranoia of Pushing a Wheelchair

When Karen made the decision that she needed a wheelchair, I think it was harder for me to face than it was for her. The idea of my wife being in a wheelchair was excruciatingly painful to me.

For years we had walked together as husband and wife. We were still husband and wife, but now I would be pushing her in a wheelchair, not walking by her side.

There is an element of pride in all this. Pushing someone in a wheelchair has a way of downsizing you. It either makes you, or breaks you. It also gives us a sense of our own mortality. The human body is a frail, delicate instrument. Sickness can strike without warning. We are as the grass of the field, and the beautiful flower, stricken and cut down before its prime.

The purchase of our first wheelchair was a bit of a shock and an eye opener for me. I simply couldn't believe a basic wheelchair was priced at five hundred dollars! It was incredible to me. I had a great deal to learn. The next chair we purchased was two thousand dollars.

The wheelchair had become a necessity for Karen. The walker was an exhausting struggle for her. Once I resigned myself to the fact that the wheelchair was going to be an inevitable part of our future, it was a relief to me too. It was painful watching Karen, struggling along, barely able to put one foot in front of the other.

I felt conspicuous and ill at ease stationed behind that chair, but I'm a grown man, with the ability to cope. It has been just as difficult for the boys, more so, because of their tender age. To walk through the mall or into a restaurant and feel the stares of the other patrons is not a pleasant experience. Zachary has commented on more than one occasion, "Daddy why do people always stare at us?" At other times he has rephrased his question to simply say, "I wish people would not stare at us."

My sons' friends for the most part have been very supportive about Karen's situation. But, I'm sure there have been instances that Jared and Zachary have had to deal with their own feelings of paranoia and embarrassment about trudging along behind their mom's wheelchair while I navigate. It is just not cool for a teenage boy to be seen in tow with his parents, especially if one of the parents is wheelchair bound.

It's human nature to empathize with those less fortunate than our selves. Frankly, I understand that it's difficult not to stare at a middle-aged man and two young boys pushing a young woman in a wheelchair. People are unaccustomed to such sights. They may be thinking to them selves, "What happened to that woman." Or, "How sad to see that family in such a difficult situation." Or they may simply be uncomfortable around sickness and infirmity. Whatever the reason, the unpleasant reality is, people are going to stare.

I have come a long way in conquering my paranoia of the wheelchair, but I would be less than truthful and the worst kind of hypocrite if I pretended that I had completely come to grips with it. The wheelchair is a constant reminder of how very ill Karen is. And frankly dear friend, that is a fact I detest. I hate the disease; and I hate the fact that she can no longer walk.

We were at a Southern Baptist Convention soon after Karen was confined to the wheelchair. It was still painfully new and uncomfortable for us. It was a strange sensation indeed, seeing old friends and colleagues. A short time after the convention, I received a telephone call from an associate who said in a very somber voice, "Glenn, I was talking to a fellow who told me he saw you at the convention and that your wife is in a wheelchair." I said simply, "Yes, she has multiple sclerosis."

If I have gleaned any thing from this experience, I have learned that I must take life one day at a time. I am less concerned now with what other people are thinking when they see me shoving and straining to position Karen in her wheelchair. And I know this is not forever. The disease may weaken Karen to the point that she is no longer able to venture out of the house.

I will trust God to see me, and my family through whatever trials and tribulations lay ahead. It's a sad, but undeniable fact that there are hundreds of thousands of persons in the United States alone, who are confined to wheelchairs. We must never lose sight of the fact that these are human beings, with the same dreams and aspirations as other people. They deserve to be treated with respect and dignity. We must be very careful to see the person, not the wheelchair, a contraption of steel and leather. Look into the invalid's eyes, you will see someone's mother or father, son or daughter, husband or wife. There but for the grace of God go I. This person is a human being, one of God's children. Never lose sight of that fact, because if we do, then we are the ones who become diminished.

Chapter 11

A Complete Change of Lifestyle

Everything was simple for Karen and I as long as she had her health. We lived a fast paced lifestyle until her diagnosis in 1990.

Karen taught school and had a ladies group she worked with at the church. Our home was always clean and well ordered; the children thrived.

Our social life was full and satisfying. Parties and gatherings of twenty to thirty people were commonplace, especially during the holiday season, when Karen made a special effort to ensure that the house was festive and inviting.

Looking back upon those days, I marvel at the ease with which Karen and I managed those functions. Admittedly, it was easier for me, than Karen. She was a wonderful hostess and went to great pains to ensure that all the preparations were handled correctly and that our guests felt welcomed and at ease in our home.

Our health is such a blessing. A blessing, unfortunately we often take for granted, until it is stripped from us.

Today having a party at our home is out of the question. Even the thought of making the preparations necessary for a single dinner guest is overwhelming. It is simply a mountain too high for us to climb.

Before Karen's illness you could expect to find us entertaining houseguests one or two weekends a month. That too, is impossible now. Karen currently spends most of her nights on the family room sofa. It is easier for her to rest there. Restless nights and frequent trips to the bathroom do not lend themselves to overnight visitors. This has been most difficult for the boys. It is a great adventure to be able to spend the night at a friend's home and then to reciprocate and have them over as your guest. It is just not practical to have the extra stress of another individual in the house. Even close friends and relatives no longer feel free to casually drop by. They realize how difficult it is to manage even an informal visit.

I never realized how much free time I had before MS entered our lives. When Karen was well and healthy I was afforded the freedom to take mission trips abroad to Africa and Brazil with no fear of the consequences to either Karen or the boys. Accepting speaking engagements out of town was never a problem. I took such luxuries very much for granted. It's a wonderful feeling to be able to pack your bags and board a plane at the drop of a hat. Karen's illness has changed all that. A line has been drawn; a boundary I must not cross. Just as an inmate knows the boundary of the prison exercise yard, so the caregiver knows how far he can journey from the invalid. They may be in trouble; they may have fallen out of the wheelchair. They are helpless and totally dependent upon you.

When I was a senior in high school I spent the week in Salyersville, Kentucky coordinating the musical portion of some worship services at a church. My pastor, Jimmy Grayson was the speaker for the week. Jimmy's wife died after a long battle with multiple sclerosis in 1993.

I had hoped that Jimmy and I would be able to spend some quality time together that week. We had only one night together in the room we shared. Jimmy confided to me that he had a sleepless night after being awakened from a dream. "Glenn, I just couldn't sleep last night. I dreamed Evelyn had fallen on the floor and couldn't get up."

As a young man of eighteen and unacquainted with illness of such magnitude I couldn't fully appreciate Jimmy's predicament. Today I understand.

If caregivers feel confined, try to imagine if you will, how much the patient suffers from this enforced captivity. They can no longer move freely in their own homes. They are totally dependent on the good will of others. A simple trip to the mall becomes an excursion that has to be planned and orchestrated in advance. This is a painful and grievous situation for a person like Karen, who was always active and vital.

When Karen was healthy and taught school her income made it possible for us to do extra things. If afforded us the opportunity to add to our savings and take a vacation in the summer. All that changed drastically when Karen was no longer able to work. The loss of income and the expenses accrued from Karen's illness has dealt us a severe financial blow.

Good health and a good spirit set us free to fly. We are able to work and provide for those we love. But what happens when our health is broken? Do we become shackled to the disease? The next time you have a virus or bad cold remember how good it felt to be well. When you are ill small problems become monumental. Just getting up in the morning may seem too great an effort.

When a debilitating disease enters the picture, our way of life changes. There is no getting around that fact. It may not be a fact we like--but it is something that has to be met head on. All one can do under such circumstances is continue to plant one foot in front of the other, and do your best. Remember we don't always get what we want in this life. An anonymous poet once said:

I asked God for strength, that I might achieve.

I was made weak, that I might learn to humbly obey.

I asked for health, that I might do greater things;

I was given infirmity, that I might do better things.

I asked for riches, that I might be happy;

I was given poverty, that I might be wise.

I asked for power that I might have the praise of men.

I was given weakness that I might feel the need of God.

I asked for all things, that I might enjoy life;

I was given life, that I might enjoy all things.

I got nothing that I asked for,

But everything I had hoped for.

I am, among all men, most richly blessed.

When the days are long and exhausting and you find yourself mourning the loss of what once was, remember, the two most important assets in anyone's life are their health, and their relationship with God. The plant that blossoms where it is planted will be transplanted. Galatians 5:7 says, "We will reap a harvest if we do not give up."

Chapter 12

What Happens to Sex?

Karen and I have been married almost twenty-four years. She was twenty-two and I was almost twenty-one on our wedding day. We have experienced some very intense, loving, sexual experiences.

From the day of our marriage until the middle of 1997 we have maintained at least the national average of sexual encounters. We could have said, "Our intimate life is over," when we received the diagnosis from Mayo Clinic. It was far from over. Looking back, there were times during those seven years when our sexual frequency increased.

Every situation and set of circumstances differ. A man who has been diagnosed with MS may suffer from impotence. Multiple sclerosis severely affects the strength in the patient's legs. This could also hamper a man's sexual performance.

I believe two people who love each other can work through these obstacles, just as Karen and I have. This may require time, patience and a lot of understanding on the part of the healthy partner. Never lose sight of the fact that the invalid may have to overcome new inhibitions about his or her body. This can be very emotionally traumatic for both the patient and the caregiver. Constant, strong assurance that everything is fine and pleasurable is a must. With a positive attitude there is no reason that both partners cannot enjoy a satisfying sex life.

Karen and I enjoyed a very satisfying sex life after she was diagnosed. I wonder how many people with MS simply give up on the idea of any kind of sexual normalcy within their marriage. How tragic for the patient or caregiver who tries to run away or neglect this wonderful aspect of the marriage relationship.

Let's be honest and realistic, there are hurdles to overcome. We are attracted to our partners because of certain physical characteristics. We look at people and say wow; they have a pretty face, nice legs, smooth skin and beautiful hair. We look at eyes, cheeks, mouths, chests, legs, and on and on. This is human nature. We are sexual creatures with sexual appetites. We are also visual creatures: Adam looked at Eve and was pleased by her physical attributes.

There are physical changes that accompany a chronic illness such as MS. These changes may develop slowly, but they will develop, it's an inevitable fact of the disease.

I remember thinking to myself, on my wedding day, as Karen walked down the aisle on her father's arm, how extraordinarily lucky I was. She was an absolute vision:

smooth, unblemished skin, black hair, and the bluest eyes I'd ever seen.

Karen is still a beauty and always will be to me. But the disease has taken a toll on her physical body.

Karen had wonderful, shapely legs. The once toned musculature of the calves and thighs has atrophied, leaving her limbs numb and wasted, the flesh discolored. Since her legs have become useless, she has had to depend on what remaining strength she has left in her hands and arms to make the transfer from wheelchair to sofa to toilet seat. In the process her legs have sustained multiple cuts and bruises, adding to their sad appearance. Her ankles and feet are permanently swollen.

Karen could have chosen to be self-conscious about the adverse physical changes that have taken place, but she chose instead to rise above any self-consciousness. She deserves a great deal of credit for that.

When Karen and I married, she was blessed with a lovely form and face, but more importantly, she was blessed with a good and generous soul. Our physical bodies will wither and age with time, but our soul which makes us truly beautiful, will never diminish. When one puts all these things into perspective, the physical changes the patient has gone through seem a very minor impediment to a satisfying sexual experience.

MS patients develop bladder problems. There is nothing quite as unsavory as walking through the front door only to be greeted by the acrid smell of urine. This is why Karen must bathe morning and evening. It is essential to the well being of the household to eliminate such unpleasant odors, and it is also essential for the physical and emotional comfort of the patient. The caregiver is asked, in this situation to go the extra mile. Bathing, dressing and caring for all the needs of the patient will fall on your shoulders. There will even be times when you may be asked to assist your wife during her menstrual cycle.

Situations such as these are not conducive to displays of passion. However, these difficulties can be overcome quite easily by planning for the moment. The care receiver needs time to prepare and get ready for the sexual encounter. Never lose sight of the fact that the patient is dependent on the care-giving spouse to assist them. This means placing them in bed and even positioning them in such a way as to make them comfortable. This requires patience, thoughtfulness, and willingness to compromise on the part of both parties. The old days of hurriedly and heatedly jumping into bed are over.

You can still approach your lovemaking with as much passion, but you will have to go slowly and methodically.

One of the toughest hurdles Karen and I have had to overcome has been the severe emotional mood swings she has experienced while under the influence of certain medications. Karen has been depressed and on occasion has experienced wild emotional outbursts of rage. There have been many days when I dreaded walking through the front door. I was never certain of the condition I would find her in.

While in the grip of depression, Karen would become verbally abusive. I didn't like this behavior, of course, but I understood what was happening to her. I was very concerned for the boys, though. She would emotionally breakdown and cry for long periods of time. The worst episodes included screaming, beating her chest, slapping her face and waving her arms wildly in the air. It was a very unnerving experience for all of us. I am very happy to report that Karen is doing much better emotionally. I credit this to the fact that she is no longer taking Beta Interferon and other drugs that may have affected her emotionally.

Making love to a person who has been verbally abusive and extremely critical of everything you are trying to do for them isn't easy. It just isn't. But you must consider the other person. If sexual intimacy is possible, and the closeness of the sex act will give the patient even a modicum of comfort, then you do it. You find a way to do it. Because of my commitment to Karen I want to accommodate her, and offer what comfort I can. She has been a wonderful partner and loyal companion. There will be times when you as a caregiver will go the second mile when you make love to your husband or wife. You will do it out of love. You will do it because your partner needs it. You will do it at times when you do not want to do it.

There may be times when you will have to turn out the lights to enjoy the sexual experience. There may be times when you will have to think about the past or the first time you made love to your partner or loving moments that you have shared together. There may be moments when you will literally have to talk yourself into the sexual experience.

We all desire intimacy, to be touched, to be treasured by another human being. Those of us who are unfortunate enough to be incapacitated because of illness are no different. We all desire intimacy with those we love. Loving a person in a sexual way is an opportunity to express and receive some of the deep emotional feeling shared by the couple.

The sexual experience will serve as a way of letting her know that you still love her and care about her needs. You are available for more than just helping her with her bath or helping her to dress in the morning. The intimacy of the sexual experience relates to the patient that they still have your heart. It reassures them that you have not emotionally left them.

It can be a time for mutual love, giving and caring. We communicate when we have sex. We communicate our feelings toward our partner. We communicate love. We communicate empathy for our partner's feelings. We communicate our desire to meet their needs.

Chapter 13

Wild Mood Swings

December 24, 1996 was like no Christmas Eve I have ever experienced. And I don't mean in the spirit of the Christmas season either.

For several years Karen's parents had been able to travel from Dayton, Ohio to attend our church's traditional Christmas Eve service. The day leading up to their arrival had been filled with tension. The boys and I had been walking on eggshells. Every missed step, no matter how slight, would induce an explosive fit of rage from Karen. I felt as though I'd been living in the midst of a natural disaster. It was like an earthquake shaking the foundations of the house every time she spoke.

Karen first experienced these extreme mood swings in the summer of 1994. We had just moved into a small apartment in Evansville, Indiana. I knew that MS could cause the patient to have emotional upsets, but these tantrums and fits of rage were incredible. It was as though Karen had been transformed into a creature I didn't know. She became an entirely different person: crazed, irrational, ranting and screaming hysterically. The slightest indiscretion, a towel out of place, a dirty dish on the kitchen counter was all the excuse she needed to lapse into a wild fit of temper. She would scream at the top of her lungs, wave her arms crazily in the air, beat her chest, slap her face and tear wildly at her clothing. Definitely not the sweet, young woman I had married.

Karen's parents had barely stepped through the door before she literally started ranting and raving. Their sad countenance told the whole story.

"What in the world is going on?" they demanded of me. "You kids need to communicate and get your act together." Karen's family believed her irrational behavior was brought on because we weren't getting along, or because the boys had done something to upset their mother. Karen's outbursts had nothing to do with our marital relationship, or the high spirits of two young boys.

The boys and I dressed and went on to the Christmas Eve service. Both boys had a part in the evening, and I of course would be leading the service as pastor. It was a wonderful service. The church was filled to capacity.

After the service Karen's father came up to me and said, "Take the kids and leave. You, nor the kids can live in this kind of environment."

Patti, Karen's sister spoke up, "Glenn how do you stand it?"

"We just hang in there and do the best we can," I replied.

"Glenn, I'm seriously thinking about going back home tonight," exclaimed her father. "I am not going to spend Christmas with her. I'm getting up in years and I can't take this anymore."

The conversation then turned to placing Karen in some kind of psychiatric unit. There was really no place available in our area that could provide the kind of care a person like Karen with her limited motor skills required.

We turned out the church lights and headed back to the house. We were fearful of going home. A man who loved his wife and two boys who loved their mother were terrified. Karen was beyond all reason. There was "no handling" her at this point. She had become a wild person. We definitely needed to do something, I just didn't know what.

When we arrived home Karen was a little more subdued. We still sensed an edge to her temperament, but the screaming and uncontrollable behavior had diminished. As the evening wore on she seemed to become quieter and more at ease. Karen's family decided not to cut short their visit and we made it through Christmas day with relative calm.

In 1989 after losing the baby, Karen experienced a deep depression. For over two years she grieved and was not herself. On more occasions than I care to remember I have heard Karen crying in the bathroom. She would sit in the bathtub talking to herself and literally sob uncontrollably for hours. She had episodes where she would become so upset and distraught I thought she was on the brink of a seizure. The muscles in her face would tremor and contort. It was quite a frightening sight to watch. These facial tremors went on for months until our family doctor prescribed a mild sedative for her. It was only a few months later that Karen was diagnosed with multiple sclerosis.

I have often wondered if Karen's lifestyle and temperament did not in some way predispose and make her more susceptible to multiple sclerosis than the average person. MS is often diagnosed after childbirth or some trauma. Karen had experienced both. MS is sometimes diagnosed when an individual has been under severe stress or the immune system is at a peak low.

Karen, remember, is a perfectionist. She would push herself to the point of exhaustion--going to bed late and rising early. She would never dream of resting until everything was done to her satisfaction. This is how she approached every aspect of her life. This stressful lifestyle and the frustration she experienced when we were unable to conceive another child must have played a significant role in weakening her immune system. I firmly believe all these factors facilitated her physical problems.

After the episode on Christmas Eve, I began to hear some disturbing news about a medication that Karen was taking. It was a steroid called prednisone. Karen had used prednisone in 1990 after the initial diagnosis was made. She had regained some of her strength while on this drug, and convinced her neurologist to prescribe it for her again.

Some of the adverse psychological side effects of prednisone can range from states of euphoria to deep profound depression. It was at this time that I also learned about the depressing properties of Beta Interferon and Avonex. These drugs were having a profoundly damaging effect upon Karen's mental health.

I did my best to convince Karen to wean herself off prednisone and Avonex. She had shown no improvement while on these medications, and if she could achieve some emotional stability I knew not only her life would improve, but so would mine, and so would the boys'.

Karen suffered a severe seizure in May 1997. Her neurologist speculated that the seizure was the result of the drug Avonex. There is no definitive proof to back up such a claim, but I felt in my heart that the Avonex was responsible for the seizure.

Slowly Karen began to accept the idea of going off the Avonex. It was a battle for her. She struggled for a week as her body slowly readjusted to the absence of the drug. Avonex is a very potent medication.

At the time of this writing Karen has been off these drugs for several months. Our home life is better. Karen is now resting better. She takes a nap. She seems much more at peace. There is a sweeter spirit to her disposition.

Our doctors never told us about the adverse side effects of the medications Karen was taking. It would have been a tremendous help if they had.

Don't wait--ask questions. Ask your doctor, how will this medication affect me? Will this medication cause crazy mood swings? Will this medication make me depressed? Will this medication cause me to act in such an irrational manner as to harm my family and home life? These are all genuine questions. And you have a right to know the answers to them.

With a disease like multiple sclerosis where the patient is so profoundly ill, desperation plays a huge roll in the decision making process. We would very likely have still tried Beta Interferon, prednisone and Avonex but we would have known what symptoms and behaviors to expect; and we might have shortened the usage of these medications. Not only would that have saved a great deal of emotional stress for my family, but also it would have made a huge difference to us financially. Receiving a statement from Berlex Laboratory for five thousand dollars is very sobering.

Even without mood altering drugs you can expect to see some very severe emotional changes from the patient. There will be days when they are seriously depressed. And you, as the caregiver, can expect to feel some depression as well. You can't see your husband or wife struggling day after day without suffering emotional pain right along with them.

Even today I will periodically hear Karen talking to herself. She speaks words of hurt, bitterness and some anger. I feel she is directing this negative energy at herself. On other occasions I feel she is talking to people who may have hurt her in the past. I think most of the time she is just talking to God, telling him how she feels.

It is very disturbing for me to hear her put herself through these emotional contortions. Berating herself, berating God and everybody else that has ever treated her in a cross or ill way.

Attitude is so vital to what we can accomplish in life. This is easy for me say. I can still walk, dress myself, play tennis, type a sermon and jump in the car and drive to the office. Not being able to do these things that we all take for granted would be an emotional hell.

Do all that is humanly possible to improve the patient's attitude. If they are still able to exercise, encourage them to stick with it. For several months Karen saw a therapist who worked with her in a heated pool. I don't think her physical condition improved, but her emotional outlook was much better. Exercise releases endorphins that send "happy signals" to our brain and body. Exercise has always contributed to a more positive productive mood from Karen. Lying on the couch all day has meant a more subdued depressed attitude.

Karen's attitude always brightens when she is able to get out of the house for a few hours. This is only natural. Before the disease she was a busy wife, mother and schoolteacher. It will be impossible to take the patient for an outing every day, but you can manage it two or perhaps three times a week. In our case I try to set aside some time on Fridays for lunch or a trip to the mall or whatever Karen wants to do. On Saturdays we may get out for a few hours and run errands.

And then there is Sunday. I love the church and being a minister, but it is still my job. This means taking Karen not only to church, but to work with me. Being a pastor is wonderfully different. But the stress of trying to greet 250 – 300 people and deliver a sermon that meets their needs after enduring the emotional surge of getting Karen up, bathed and dressed and then transported is an experience--to say the least.

In the midst of it all, keep these items in mind when dealing with the emotions of your sick loved one. You are a good, caring person or you wouldn't take the time to read this book. Because you do care, journey on with me.

Chapter 14

Coping With the Suicidal Threats of the Patient

I thought about entitling this chapter, "The Suicidal Tendencies of the Patient," but in Karen's case and in the case of many chronically ill patients, it has gone beyond the "tendency" stage. Karen has on numerous occasions threatened to take her own life. Generally, these suicidal threats have occurred when she was in the throws of a serious depression, or experiencing wild irrational mood swings.

There are several schools of thought about people who commit suicide. There is the theory that if a person talks about killing him or herself, they should not be taken seriously; it is merely a cry for help and attention. Another theory holds that the person who seriously intends to commit suicide will forewarn no one. And lastly, the next theory states that both of the above are untrustworthy.

I had a first cousin that committed suicide. He was a wonderful young man: smart, talented and handsome, but he'd had a hard life growing up. After several years of marriage his wife left him for another man. The break-up of his marriage was more than he could cope with. I have been told that he talked of suicide with his mother. Several days before he killed himself, he asked his mother if she would care for his children if anything were to happen to him. She was shocked, but assured him she would. A few days later he went out into a field not too far from his house and shot himself.

A young lady whose house I used to visit as a child with my parents became distraught and took her life in her car. A pistol was found beside her dead body along with a good-bye letter. No one knew she had been thinking about ending her life.

In 1991, I was called one Sunday morning to a family's house in Pikeville because their beautiful nineteen-year-old daughter had been found dead in the front seat of her car. The pistol that the girl apparently carried in her car was found beside her. It came as a total shock to the family and community that this beautiful, healthy young college student had taken her life. There had never been any conversation or warning about suicide. She seemingly had everything going for her.

As you can see from these examples there are no hard and fast rules when it comes to second-guessing how someone who is suicidal will react. My cousin openly discussed his feelings about suicide, while the other two cases came as a complete shock to family and friends.

Suicidal thoughts may be triggered by deep depression. Someone may contemplate taking his or her life after a traumatic loss. In most circumstances, the person experiences a profound sense of hopelessness and worthlessness. They see no other way out of whatever difficulties may be plaguing them, so they opt for suicide.

A friend of mine, who is a minister, went through a divorce. For a period of time, he was without employment and away from his children. "I actually thought about taking my life," he confided. He went on, "I saw no life ahead for me. I knew no church would hire me because of my divorce. I had nothing left to give my children and it seemed everyone had turned against me. I had hit rock bottom. I just couldn't see any way out."

Somehow he managed to come to terms with his feelings of hopelessness and despair, and continued on with his life. Today he is remarried and once again pastoring a church.

If I committed suicide it would be like me saying to my two boys who are at home and in school, "To hell with you. Take care of yourselves. I don't give a flip about what happens to you."

I don't think many suicide victims actually see their death this way. Sadly they lose sight of how devastating their death will be to those who love them and are left behind. It is the surviving spouse who is left to ponder, "What could I have done differently?" The children are left to spend their lives wondering, "Why did daddy or mommy leave me?"

I have heard many testify that suicide is an extremely selfish act, perpetuated by individuals who care only for themselves and their pain. But what of the person whose mind is so clouded, and his or her reasoning processes so distorted by drugs that they are unable to come to terms with feelings of hopelessness and self-loathing? What of the individual who has lived with clinical depression for years and because of a chemical imbalance in the brain is simply unable to see the light at the end of the tunnel? I refuse to call these unfortunate people selfish.

What do you do when someone is talking about taking his or her own life? You take them very seriously, and don't ignore it. You listen to what they are saying and act accordingly. If they are talking about taking an overdose, then you pay attention to the medicine bottles. The time may come when you the caregiver, must dispense all medications to the patient. If you must be away from home during the day, then have the exact dosage of all medications set out for them.

Tell the patient's family. In our case I made it a point to convey to Karen's family what she was talking about. This is a problem no one should have to face alone. You need just as much support and encouragement as does the patient.

Talk to someone outside your immediate family about the suicide threats. This can be close friends or a professional counselor.

By all means report the suicide threats to the patient's doctor. He may want to adjust levels of medication or prescribe an anti-depressant to help the care receiver through this difficult time.

Listen to the patient. Sometimes they are merely crying out for attention. They are sick and lonely and troubled and life is hard for them. Try to find out what has brought on these feelings of suicide. Ask what you can do to help ease their mind. Be prepared to hear every kind of answer under the sun. When a person is suicidal they are not rational.

Do whatever is necessary to keep the patient safe. Have someone in the family or close friend stay in touch during the day when you are at work.

If someone really wants to end their own life, they can find a way. All we can do is our best.

Karen has on many occasions talked about ending her life. If such a thing were to actually occur, it would be devastating to our family. We love Karen.

We have been married for over twenty-four years. You cannot spend twenty-four years of your life with someone, have children with that person and go through what we have without developing deep, lasting, emotional ties.

She continues to make a tremendous contribution to our family. Three and sometimes four nights a week Karen can be found sitting at our kitchen table with Jared and Zachary going over homework assignments.

I cannot really document the first time Karen said she was going to end her life. I think it was probably in 1993. We had moved into a large house in Louisa, Kentucky with a double car garage. Karen, during a very emotional mood swing said she was tired of watching her health dissipate. She announced she had figured out a way to painlessly take her life.

I honestly had no clue what she was talking about. I later found out her plan was to lock the garage doors, start one of the cars and simply wait until the level of carbon monoxide became lethal.

On New Years Eve, 1996, Karen had a panic attack like no other panic attack she has ever suffered. Karen was completely out of control, even in the presence of one of her best friends. Usually during one of these episodes Karen could be counted on to get her emotions in check in the presence of someone outside the immediate family. She was beyond that.

Every move she made that evening terrified her. For hours that night she was afraid she was falling out of her chair. "Help me, help me," she would call out to me. "I am falling." She grasped the arms of her chair in a state of absolute panic.

While her friend was with us in our family room, Karen leaned over and whispered in my ear, "Glenn I want you to call that doctor."

"What doctor are you talking about? Who would you like me to call?" I asked.

"I want you to call that doctor I have heard about on the television. You know, Dr. Kevorkian."

I looked at our friend and tried to laugh. "Honey, we are not calling Dr. Kevorkian. Everything will be all right. I will take you to the hospital if you would be willing to go."

"Oh no I don't want to go to the hospital," she replied.

Karen eventually began to calm down. However, it was almost eleven o'clock that night before her friend felt comfortable enough to go home. Karen finally fell into an exhausted sleep. The next morning she was fine and acted as though nothing had happened the night before.

On other occasions Karen has talked about taking an overdose. This was a constant source of worry for me. Karen had at her disposal many medications that could have proven fatal if taken in excess. I never knew if Karen's self-destructive talk was just a cry for help or if she seriously intended to end her life. For months I worried whenever I came home and found Karen in a deep sleep that maybe she'd taken too much medication.

The fear and trepidation of coming home and finding my wife dead of her own hand lasted for almost three years. Since about the middle of 1997 there has been a greater sense of peace and calm around our home. Karen seems to have worked through her thoughts of suicide. We all hope and pray for her daily, that she can remain strong and steadfast.

Chapter 15

Coping with Stress

Are you going to survive all this? Caring for someone on a daily basis is a long difficult road. It's a lonely road. Are you feeling the effects of it? It's not easy. Caring for someone who is becoming as helpless as a baby costs us. The general day to day care of the patient along with all the demands placed upon you to be ready and available at all times is stressful, to say the least. There is no time or energy left for anything else. Depending on how we handle this stress, it will either make us, or break us.

In this chapter I want to look at ways the caregiver can handle some of the inevitable stress. If you do not learn to manage stress, it will send you to your grave long before the loved one you're caring for.

You must have a spiritual connection to make it on this journey. I realize not everyone reading this book will be a Christian. I can only say that without my heavenly Father to look to and depend upon, I would never have survived the ordeal, thus far.

I realize that there are many of you reading this chapter, who are hurt and disillusioned. You may be asking yourselves the question, "Why would a loving heavenly Father place such burdens upon his children?" I don't know. I do know that God allows tragedy in this world. From the very beginning of time the human race has suffered heartache. The Bible chronicles the trials of Job, war and pestilence and the division of families. But in the midst of the chaos is God's love. The Bible says God is love. Would a loving God allow MS? Yes he does and will continue to do so. Will He give you the strength and courage to see you through it? Yes, He will. The Bible says, "Cast all your anxiety on him because he cares for you." (I Peter 5:7).

There is a tremendous sense of relief in being able to place our burdens in God's hands. There is strength and power in meditation. Begin each day if only for five or ten minutes focusing your thoughts on God's help. This is vital to your sense of well-being. In the afternoon or evening, when you are able to spare a few minutes, give thanks to God for seeing you through yet another day. This will help you to sleep at night. Don't take your troubles to bed. Don't wrestle all night with your worries and fears. Put these problems in God's hands.

Within every person there is an internal empty space that cries out to be filled. People try filling it with relationships, work, success, alcohol, sex, drugs, entertainment and on and on. These pleasures offer some sense of gratification, but they will never bring one inner peace. There is a part of us that cries out to be filled by a peace that passes all understanding. This peace is attained by our relationship with God through His Son Jesus Christ.

You will need someone to talk to. I cannot overstate the importance of finding someone you can trust to periodically share with. You may find this a difficult task. It is not easy to find a support group for caregivers. Try to find others who are going through what you are, or who have experienced care giving. Check with your local hospital. Be a pest. Check with the hospital chaplain. Ask him to put you in touch with caregivers in similar situations. Ask your doctor about support groups.

The Internet can be a good and positive tool. You might consider starting a chat room for caregivers. You may be surprised by the shear number of people, who just like you, are looking for someone to share with. Develop these friendships slowly and with caution. Be wary of giving out too much personal information, such as your real name and address.

If the Internet does not appeal to you, or if you prefer the one to one interaction of speaking to someone personally, consider talking to a trusted friend, pastor, or professional counselor. Choose your confidants carefully. If you want what you say to be held in strictest confidence, talking about your troubles to your Sunday school class or a civic group would be unwise.

If you are a good organization person, and time permitting, you might consider starting your own support group to meet at your church, community center or in your home. You will need to run an advertisement in your local paper and post notices on several church and hospital bulletin boards. This extra effort will pay off when you find other people in your community to share your feelings with. Don't go for five, ten, or twenty years carrying this burden in your heart without finding a sympathetic listener.

You will need rest. Taking care of someone else is physically exhausting. Our bodies only function well when rested. In my case I am the daddy of two active boys, a pastor of a growing suburban church and a caregiver to a sick wife. Somewhere I have to sneak some rest in.

When you are tired and need a nap then take one. Try to go to bed about the same time every night and rise the same time every morning. Schedules are important to our biological clock. You will be better able to cope with all that is demanded of you during the day if you give your body what it needs.

Along with proper rest comes good eating habits and exercise. I feel very strongly about the value of good nutrition and exercise, so strongly that I devoted chapter 16 to the subject.

Before I leave this chapter, I want to admonish the reader to be very careful how you use your tongue. Loud verbal negative statements are seldom forgotten.

I don't scream or raise my voice to Karen. I never have and I never will. There have been many occasions when I have felt like screaming and railing at her.

When negative, hurtful words are uttered, they can never be retracted. You can say, "I'm sorry," until you're blue in the face. Life is difficult and stressful enough without adding regret to your list of problems.

I know dear friends; the road we travel seems incredibly hard and treacherous. Someday we will be on the other side of this life. I believe at that point we will look back and understand it much better. I will be able to understand why Karen was stricken with MS. I will have an understanding of how our suffering was used for good to help others in their journey. That is in the future. We live in the present. Right now it is hard, very hard. But someday soon, we will see and understand all.

Chapter 16

Exercise

Exercise is a must for the caregiver. I cannot emphasize that strongly enough. There is nothing quite like it for neutralizing the stress and tensions of the day. You will sleep better at night, feel better, look better and be a calmer and happier person. Now, don't you deserve that?

Exercise has always been important to me. Growing up in Appalachia meant seclusion. My social life was somewhat limited by today's standards. Until I was fifteen years old my grandparents operated a grocery store. This provided a tremendous social outlet for me. People came and went. My mother's brothers and sisters and their children often spent afternoons sitting around the store chatting.

Besides this I had access to a basketball goal in the cow pasture about a hundred yards from our house. Playing on a dirt court in a cow pasture presented some challenges. For one, the basketball court was a favorite "rest stop" for the cattle. This meant clearing a path on the court before I could begin my practice shots. And no matter how carefully I tried, I always neglected that one cow pile at the edge of the court.

Of course that was exactly where the ball would inevitably land.

There was seldom a day from the time I was six years old, until I was fourteen that I didn't shoot hoops on that dirt court. Most of the time I would return home with dirty hands and soaked with sweat. But after an hour of giving it my all, I always felt so much better.

Cycling was another form of exercise I enjoyed as a boy. My parents bought me a bicycle when I was about seven years old. By the time I was ten or eleven years old it had become my means of escape. My friends and I would all get together and ride our bikes three or four miles every day up and down Milo Road. I attribute my leanness to my active lifestyle. My senior year of high school I was 6'3 and 185 pounds.

There was a creek that ran in front of my house. As a kid I loved wading in that creek. There were even a couple of water holes deep enough to swim in. It was great fun and a tremendous way of letting off steam.

Being raised in Appalachia also meant growing up among the hills. I loved wandering the hills and valleys. There was never any danger in our area of running into strangers or wild animals. It was a great way to get away from your problems.

Looking back I realize how important basketball, cycling, swimming and the hills of Appalachia were to me. I found happiness and a feeling of fulfillment as a boy by exercising and having hobbies that benefited my body and spirit.

There is an emotional numbing to care giving. There are many days when it seems like your life is on a perpetual treadmill. Your main concern for the day may be to ensure the patient is bathed, dressed, fed, taken out of the house for a joy ride and conversed with.

This leaves little time for your own personal needs. You consider yourself lucky to be able to squeeze in a few minutes for a shower. Maybe there is a favorite television program you enjoy so you try to watch it. The grass needs mowed so you mow the grass and cut the weeds. There is always laundry to be done. The list is endless.

Chances are the whole idea of exercise is a joke to you. You're probably chuckling right now, if you haven't already skipped this chapter. Or perhaps you'd rather hear me talk about what a lousy hand of cards we've been dealt. Do you just want to sit and pout about being a caregiver? It rains on the just and unjust alike, my friend. We all have to play with the hand we've been dealt, whether we like the cards or not.

And one of the ways to make the best of a tough situation is through exercise.

You must find a way to exercise. Whether you exercise in your home or at a gym, you need an exercise program that will allow you to work up a good sweat three or four times a week for at least thirty minutes. You need this release. Exercise provides a wonderful escape.

Cardiovascular exercise may be termed aerobic exercise. A person who runs, plays basketball or jumps rope is engaging in aerobic exercise. An aerobic workout should stimulate the heart to pump faster and maintain that heart rate for at least twenty minutes.

Aerobics looked a little scary to me when I watched my first class at a health club in Lexington, Kentucky. Most of the aerobics classes I have attended since that time have been set to upbeat popular music. The movements such as jumping jacks, push-ups and running in place make for a phenomenal workout. One more advantage to an aerobics class, is convenience. It's never too hot or too cold to exercise, which is not always the case in mid-August or mid-January.

I attend a lot of aerobic classes at a local gym. I go and work out hard. I holler and scream and just have a wonderful time. I get a high from it. I'm serious. Sometimes by the middle of the class I find myself laughing uncontrollably.

Exercise releases endorphins to the brain, which alters our mood. We feel more peaceful and happy.

I may go to a class and feel lousy and may have even thought about not doing the class. I start working and moving and exercising and it's amazing how my disposition begins to change. If I have been drinking coffee during the day or have eaten junk food exercise has a way of purging my body. The workout also seems to purge my mind. I may have had a difficult day with Karen or the people I work with, but by the end of my exercise routine I have a clean feeling. I am then able to go home and be a better caregiver to Karen.

If a structured aerobics class is not to your liking, you may take advantage of treadmills, stationary bicycles and a variety of other exercise equipment that any reputable health club should have on the premises. Never be hesitant about asking one of the club staff to demonstrate the proper uses of these machines. If you're going to exercise, you want to ensure that you're receiving the maximum benefits from your workout, plus knowing the correct way to use the exercise equipment will eliminate strained muscles and injuries.

As we grow older our muscle mass and bone density begins to diminish. Our level of strength deteriorates. A wonderful way to maintain muscle tone and strength is by lifting weights.

Free weights can be found at almost any health club. As the name implies, free weights are not connected to any chains or pulleys. If a weight is labeled twenty pounds, then it is up to your muscles to lift that twenty-pound weight. Again I cannot over emphasize the importance of learning the correct procedure for lifting free weights from a member of the club staff. You will also be introduced to many weight machines that operate using a system of chains and pulleys. These too when used properly will benefit muscle tone and help you maintain the strength and stamina needed in your every day life as a caregiver.

As Karen's condition has continued to deteriorate I have had less and less time to go to the gym. I think the average caregiver can easily identify with this problem.

Not only can time be a factor, but guilt also plays a role in how much time caregivers feel they should be away from the patient in pursuit of their own lives and interests. Don't let guilt rule your life--this is crazy!

You must give yourself permission to go on with life. It is simply a case of making a decision to do something that will benefit you both in mind and body. No one else will tell you to take care of yourself. There could even be some resentment from family and peers. You must learn to ignore them. After all friend, if your health goes--then who will take care of your loved one, and who will take care of you?

I live in the real world, and I know that most caregivers are strapped for cash. Even those of us fortunate enough to have some medical insurance are still faced with deductibles and extras that insurance companies refuse to reimburse.

A health club, when considering the whole picture, is one of the smartest financial investments you can make. Shop around; investigate the different health clubs in your area. I think you'll be pleasantly surprised. In my town, health club fees range from seventeen dollars per month, all the way to one hundred dollars per month.

You've checked out all the health clubs in your area, you've weighed the pros and cons, but for whatever reason, you simply can't manage it, then be creative. You can exercise in your home or jog around the block. But do something. If you are a caregiver who has outside employment, you may have to get up a little earlier to exercise, or fit your routine in before you go home for the day. Or better yet, exercise on your lunch hour. You will be avoiding those noontime calories, plus you will be more alert and energized.

It is common today to purchase exercise machines: treadmills, stationary bicycles, Stairmasters, I could go on and on, the list is endless. Exercise machines are great, unless they become a convenient place to hang clothes. And if money is a consideration, which it is for most of us, remember you can easily tie up to two thousand dollars in a treadmill alone.

The average caregiver is strapped for cash. Utilize the subdivision or country road where you live. Take walks or develop the ability to jog. Do jumping jacks in front of the television while watching an exercise program. Develop ways to exercise in the back yard or do sit ups, pushups and other exercises that can be done in the home.

Before closing this chapter, let me reiterate the importance of taking care of yourself. Exercise isn't the only answer to maintaining good health and a positive outlook on life, but it's definitely part of the answer. The very fact that you are taking charge of your body, and giving it what it needs, will make you a better caregiver.

Chapter 17

Be Careful About What You Eat

Since we are talking about exercise and fitness it behooves me to say a word about nutrition. You can exercise your day away and still become overweight and feel tired and sluggish.

I must stop here, and confess that I speak from personal experience. I have been through this stage more than once. I would rationalize, "Okay, I worked out for forty minutes. My heart pumped hard. I worked up a good sweat." And then I would head for the kitchen and a wedge of pie. Or, I would use the same rationale for a bowl of ice cream right before bedtime.

My profession as a minister keeps me in constant danger. Well perhaps not literally in danger, it would be better to say temptation. Our church is known for hosting some terrific potluck dinners. Plus I have a lot of wonderful people in my life that frequently extend breakfast and luncheon invitations. It is so easy to simply say, eat, drink and be merry. That attitude added an extra fifteen pounds to my waistline.

While it is certainly true that exercising burns off calories you cannot continue to fudge on foods that are high in fat and sugar content without it eventually catching up to you. There has never been an exercise routine, no matter how strenuous, that you cannot out eat.

For example, let's say you stop by your favorite fast food restaurant and order a double cheeseburger, large fries, and a large chocolate shake. You are consuming approximately one thousand calories and fifty grams of fat.

So, to soothe your conscience and justify this high calorie, high fat lunch you say to yourself, "Well, I'll go to the gym tonight and work it off." To burn off a thousand calories you would have to exercise hard for at least ninety minutes. I have burned off a thousand calories on the Stairmaster, and let me assure you, when the workout is over I am exhausted and drenched with sweat.

It is much easier and far more productive to simply eat better and eat in moderation. Meals consisting of greasy hamburgers and steak will make you fat and sluggish. You don't need that. You have enough to contend with, as it is. The very fact that you have someone in your household that requires your constant care and attention is a heavy load. Why would you want to add the extra burden of thirty unnecessary pounds to that load?

We are what we eat. If you eat pizza and cheeseburgers and fried foods you are going to feel lousy. I know it isn't easy to eliminate these foods from your diet, and you can still treat yourself occasionally, but you can't continue to fuel your body with junk and not suffer the consequences--weight gain.

I am quite honest about the fact that on any given night you may see me bringing fast food home for dinner. If fast food is on the agenda, look for a restaurant that serves grilled chicken or a baked potato or salad. The grilled chicken sandwich, plain of course, will only have about three hundred to three hundred fifty calories and may contain around seven grams of fat. Ask for water, or a caffeine free diet soda. Try to hold the toppings to a minimum on your baked potato. Instead of a thousand calories, you have reduced that number to around six hundred calories--a much more manageable number of calories to burn off at your workout.

Watch out for large amounts of caffeine. I recommend limiting your coffee consumption to less than five cups a day. This may be difficult in the beginning. I love to drink coffee. There is nothing I like better than a big cookie and a cup of coffee. The rush of sugar and caffeine instantly perks me up, but on the down side, it can just as quickly let you crash, feeling depleted and sluggish. I know that a cup of coffee after 2:00 p.m. is a mistake I will pay for with a sleepless night.

Not only is your diet crucial to your health and well-being, but the patient will benefit too. Nutrition is an important element in the management of MS. Karen has been in a wheelchair for almost five years. At the present time she weighs one hundred twenty pounds and is still able to wear the same clothing she did before she became dependent upon her wheelchair. This is a remarkable feat. Karen is very careful to watch portions and only occasionally indulges in candy and fried foods.

I personally feel vitamins are vital to the caregiver. I take a chewable adult vitamin C tablet and a multi-vitamin tablet every day. And yes they make chewable vitamins for adults. It's just more fun to chew a good tasting tablet than gulping one down with a sip of water. No matter how good our intentions, there are days when we do not get enough of what we need from the foods we eat. The vitamins seem to give me that little extra boost I need to complete my day. If I don't get that nap in the afternoon, the vitamins seem to keep me going until my ten-thirty bedtime.

Check with your doctor before beginning any kind of rigorous diet or exercise program. Always begin slowly and pace yourself. You don't have to get it all done in a day or a week or the first month.

Proper nutrition and moderate exercise will enhance your journey as a caregiver. Anything you can do to improve your own self-image will lighten the load of caring for your sick loved one.

Chapter 18

You Must Have A Life

Taking care of someone is surely a life of love, dedication and service. It is quite true that when we go out of our way to fulfill the needs of another person, then our lives are richer for it. There is only one problem with this. Taking care of someone can become your life. I mean quite literally that you lose your life and self-identity to the care receiver.

Total dedication with no thought about yourself or your future may be all right for a few months. You may be able to do it for a few years. But the day will come when you wake up one morning and look around and realize you've lost yourself. Every ounce of energy and creativity has gone into caring for your sick wife, husband or child. It isn't long after that realization before a certain amount of resentment toward the patient starts to color your perspective.

Do you think that's harsh--that someone could actually resent another person who is desperately ill and confined to a wheelchair? You can't know what it means to be on call twenty-four hours a day, seven days a week, unless you've done it. Please don't judge me, but try if you can to understand.

The patient you are caring for is in need of help. They are dependent upon you for everything. They soon lose touch with how much they were doing before becoming ill. It's easy to forget about the demands of work and hectic schedules and what it takes to really keep everything going, when you are confined to your house, and a wheelchair.

So, there are questions like, "What do you have to do today? Where have you been so long? Why do you leave the house so early?" In Karen's case, she knows she is sick. She knows we love her and she knows we are going to take care of her.

There is a lot of leverage in that kind of knowledge. Even so, her demands and expectations are sometimes unrealistic. It would be very easy for my sons and I to do nothing but carry out Karen's wishes. Let me say that we want to do all we can to make her as comfortable and as happy as possible. But does that mean that my son never goes on a scout trip? Does this mean that my children and I never do anything as father and sons?

It isn't easy to walk out the door and leave the patient behind. Karen has always resented it, and I understand her feelings. It is heartbreaking not to be involved as thoroughly in her children's lives, as she would like. This has always been very tough for me, and I know it will be tough for you as a caregiver to make the decision, that yes, there are going to be times when you will have to go on with your life and exclude the patient. But you have to do it.

I had two choices. I could go on living, or I could crawl into that wheelchair with Karen and die too. I have chosen to live and continue forward with my life. I have suffered terrible pangs of guilt because I still have dreams and aspirations for my life. It's taken a lot of time and prayer for me to overcome that guilt. But it is essential for me, just as it is for you, to keep your dreams in front of you. A part of my dream is that Karen will get better. I have prayed almost without ceasing for a miracle.

I want to ask you this very important question and I want you to answer it truthfully. What is your dream? Yes, you want your loved one to be better and for all this to be behind you. Life would be wonderful again if that were to happen. But what if it doesn't happen? What if your husband or wife is sick and homebound for five, ten or more years? What if they are sick the rest of your life? What then?

You had a dream for your life once, I know you did. Did you lose it? Where did you lose it? Did you lose it in a hospital room? Did you lose it in a doctor's office? Did you lose it changing your wife's underpants? Did you lose your dream when you were being lambasted with disapproval? Did you lose your dream after an exhausting day trying to be all things to all people, and failing?

It's easy to give up and cast all dreams and hopes for the future aside. You live only for the present, hoping just to make it through one more day. Do you have children? You must force yourself to think past the moment and into the future for them.

Do great things in spite of your circumstances. Have you ever heard that before? "I'm doing good to make it under the circumstances," you say. Yes, I know we travel a hard road, but let me ask you this. When have our circumstances ever been perfect? When has life ever been without a hurdle to jump or a puddle to cross? I know sometimes the hurdles are mountains and the puddles are oceans. But with God's help and guidance you can devise a way to make these seemingly impossible obstacles manageable. Be a blessing to your loved one and a blessing to all whose lives you touch.

I love to write and writing is something I can do almost anywhere. It wasn't easy, under the circumstances, to write this book, but I did it. And you can fulfill your dreams too.

If you are forced to be at home around the clock with the patient, look for opportunities that will allow you to work at home. This is the age of the computer. It is amazing how much business is conducted over the Internet. Many businesses need people who can do secretarial work and place telephone calls. Much of this could be done from your home. I've just scratched the surface. The opportunities are endless if we will only let ourselves dream and explore the possibilities.

Don't stop living because someone you love is ill. This helps no one. Make the most of your life. Do great things in spite of your circumstances and utilize your opportunities. Be a good steward to your loved one, and just as importantly, be a good steward to yourself.

Chapter 19

Let Others Help

I would never have dreamed of having someone in our house helping Karen or doing anything for our family. The idea of needing someone to help bathe my wife or help with laundry was completely out of my realm of thinking.

When Karen was diagnosed with MS, I decided that I would be there to help her with whatever she needed. I believe this is how many caregivers feel in the beginning. But let me tell you, you can't do it all. You must accept help.

This was tough. I went through a very negative time, and did a lot of soul searching. Relying on others is difficult; I know it's been a difficult transition for me. I wanted to be there to care for Karen all the time. But it just wasn't possible. So I had to face the unpleasant fact that if I didn't graciously accept the help that was offered, Karen would be the one to suffer and this was totally unacceptable to me.

I am a very independent and private person. I don't particularly enjoy having things done for me. I don't mind paying somebody to mow the lawn or wash the windows, but acts of charity although much appreciated, can also be humbling.

Don't let false pride hamper you. So many times I have been approached by members of my congregation, who will earnestly ask, "What can I do to help your family? What can I do to help Karen?" And so many times, far too numerous to count I have said, "Nothing." I have got to stop that! And if you're guilty of saying the same thing, then you must learn to stop too. That is insane. The sane thing to do when asked these questions is jump in and say, "Well, at about noon tomorrow you could come by the house. I have some cold cuts in the refrigerator and you can make yourself and Karen a sandwich."

Just knowing that I don't have to stop in the middle of my day to rush home and fix lunch for Karen is a tremendous help, but more importantly having someone in the house to talk to for an hour or two is great for Karen's morale.

Karen spends a great deal of time alone. And because of this she has felt ignored and lonely. Being in the house all day means boredom. There is television and the telephone is always near by, but it has its limitations. What she really craves is someone to talk to.

As a pastor, much of my day is spent listening to other people, usually listening to their problems. Like every other normal American I have days when I need to come home from work and lie down on the couch and unwind. Being bombarded with requests and the patient's need to talk as soon as you walk through the front door is draining and unhealthy.

I can always tell when Karen has had a friend over. Having someone drop by the house for a thirty-minute visit makes a huge difference in her attitude. She is much more content and far less needy of attention. She has had the opportunity to converse with someone who values her enough to set aside time just to talk.

A lady from our church picks Karen up for a Bible study almost every Tuesday. She arrives and helps Karen into her car, takes her to Bible study and then to lunch. It's a great break for Karen and something she looks forward to each week. It not only provides her an outing, but she has the opportunity to be with other ladies.

One lady in our church on several occasions has picked Karen up just to go to the mall. It requires helping her to dress and if circumstances dictate helping her in the lady's room. Why would I refuse help from these wonderful people and deny Karen something that is so emotionally healthy?

People want and need to help. Please, let them. Your family and friends know you're only human. We all have limitations. There is only so much one person can do alone. I don't know of anyone who will give you a badge for doing it all. You may be on some kind of noble mission to impress people with how much stress you can handle and how efficiently you manage to care for your loved one. But no one is really impressed. They may be impressed by your good attitude. Your positive spirit may inspire them. But there will be times when they will wonder why you expend so much energy putting up a front. Why won't you let people help you?

If a retired person you know wants to volunteer some time to help take the patient out for a drive, let them. If someone offers to help with some cleaning or laundry, let them. If a neighbor drops by at dinnertime with a casserole, accept it graciously. Don't turn down anything that is helpful to the patient and in turn can lighten your burden as a caregiver.

Every situation is different. And the kind of care each patient needs is very individualized. Not everyone who offers their assistance is able to handle the stress and complications of transporting someone like Karen.

I have encountered people who were very insistent about wanting to lend a helping hand. They meant well, but tried and tired quickly. I understand. The average person simply doesn't know what is involved in caring for someone in a wheelchair. They don't realize that Karen must be literally picked up and placed in the car. She needs help with undressing and dressing when she goes to the bathroom.

Managing a wheelchair is a major task within itself. Wheelchairs are painful. They hurt when you run into them. They are painful when the wheels run over your toes. It's easy to get your fingers pinched when folding and unfolding the chair, which is excruciatingly painful. The wheelchair may or may not fit into the trunk of the car.

When a volunteer discovers what an undertaking it is to care for someone in a wheelchair for a day, many have had second thoughts. I am truly amazed at the faithfulness of our friends who continue almost weekly to come back time after time to help Karen.

As I stated, every case is different and unique. For example, at the time of this writing my mother is almost eighty-two years old. She has led a very active and productive life. But sometimes she forgets and takes too much medication. Case in point, she took some over the counter cold medication, which reacted adversely with medication that she takes to lower her blood pressure, resulting in a week's stay at the hospital.

I am very fortunate to have two sisters and one brother who still live close to Mom and Dad. My sisters are wonderful about looking in on my parents and running errands. Not too long ago both my parents had to be hospitalized. I wanted so much to be able to go to them, but because of Karen's situation, I simply couldn't leave.

I can't tell you how grateful I am to have the help of my brothers and sisters. I know I can rely upon them to take care of our parents in a kind and loving way. I would never dream of begrudging their help. So why would I begrudge our friends and neighbors when out of love they want to help Karen?

Perhaps your problem is not one of misplaced pride, or too much self-reliance. If you are in need of help but don't know where to look, here are some options for you to check into.

Start by checking the Yellow Pages in your telephone book for Home Health Care Agencies. Call the agencies, they will be glad to find out for you what Medicare will cover.

Churches and civic organizations are another excellent source of help. Call the pastor of a local church and ask, "Pastor, do you know of a Sunday school class that would like a project? I really need some help caring for my sick mother, father, child or spouse. Would you speak to one of the adult teachers about sharing our situation with their class?" I can't promise what kind of reception you will receive, but I think you will eventually have some help.

Check with the non-profit organizations in your community. If you are caring for someone with Alzheimer's, I would call the Alzheimer's Society. They will have the inside track on public services in your community where you may solicit help. At the very least they will be able to furnish a list of telephone numbers for you to call.

Your doctor or hospital should have a list of support groups in your area. If there is an Alzheimer's or multiple sclerosis support group they may know of someone who is looking for part-time employment as a caregiver.

You may consider placing an advertisement in your local newspaper. This must be done with great care. Make sure you ask for references from all responders and check out their references with a fine toothcomb. You can't be too careful.

It's a lonely journey, especially if you're trying to carry the burden alone. You love the person you're caring for. You love your parent. You love your child. You love your wife or husband. Because you love them, let others help.

Chapter 20

What People Expect of You as a Caregiver

Maybe you have had days when you felt tremendous expectations from everybody. You felt expectations from the loved one you care for. You felt expectations from other family members. You felt expectations from friends and even neighbors. Expectations are those pressures we feel about our circumstances, whether real or imagined.

Nobody likes to function under pressure. There are times, however, when pressure is a good and necessary thing. A rubber band is worthless unless it is tense. A tea bag is useless unless it is in hot water. Flowers don't grow without some rain. We don't achieve and move forward without goals and the ambition to see those goals through to the end. Sometimes pressure has a way of bringing out the very best in us.

The NCAA basketball champions for 1998 were the University of Kentucky Wildcats. They became known as the "Comeback Cats." Never in the history of the NCAA has a team fought back the way they did. Each game it looked as though they would be defeated, but against all odds they forged ahead and experienced victory.

A young woman who joined our church talked about her experiences of caring for her terminally ill husband who suffered from kidney cancer. Reflecting back on the situation she was able to say, "I feel like I'm a better person having gone through that. It has made me appreciate the life I have today."

Just as pressure can be the impetus we need to strive and achieve; life's expectations can also spur us on to rise above our circumstances. For example, it is expected that I will take care of my wife and children. It is expected that I will do this with a smile on my face and a sunny disposition. I am expected to orchestrate the day to day running of our household, which includes everything from dressing and bathing Karen, to getting the boys off to school, to cooking dinner and everything else in between. Plus I am expected to have gainful employment.

But what happens if you as the caregiver decide one day that you're tired and you don't want to rise to the occasion. Does that make you a bad person? No, I think that makes you human.

Let's talk about some of those expectations. I am expected to take care of my wife and family. And without question that is what I have done and will continue to do. Does that mean it's been an easy adjustment? Absolutely not.

When I married Karen I never dreamed she would be diagnosed with MS. The fact that she's sick and in a wheelchair does not change our love or our marriage relationship. But it does change the scenario of our lives.

There have been days when I wanted to throw my hands up in despair and quit; turn my back on the whole affair and leave. But I don't, I stay and do my best. Some days my best seems pitifully little and I feel as much like a failure as a man can. But dear friends, I can't overemphasize this point enough--all anyone can expect of you, and all you can expect from yourself, is your best.

You are not a machine. Machines can operate with maintenance and the flip of a switch. When a machine breaks down then a new part replaces the broken one and the machine continues. Or, the machine is replaced with a new model. We require maintenance too: proper rest, nutrition, exercise and most importantly, affirmation. Unlike machines we have emotions. We have energy levels that can be depleted. Machines don't get lonely, frustrated and need support groups. They don't have to deal with life's expectations. They don't have the fear of failure. They just function.

I love Karen very much. I would never want to do anything but help her because she is my wife and I care for her deeply. But while I feel love for her, I also feel committed and obligated. At one point or another in your personal journey as a caregiver you will experience one or all three of these emotions. The fact that you are caring for someone out of commitment or even obligation does not mean you do not love them. It is because you love them that you are committed and obligated to care for them.

Therefore, each day and night you do your best. Sometimes I don't want to be a caregiver. And then I see my wife who I love, the mother of my children, and I think of all the things we have experienced and I know that I must find a way to keep going, to survive. Sometimes it is love that sustains me, sometimes it is commitment, and sometimes it is a sense of sheer obligation.

People say to me, "I don't see how you are doing it. I don't think I could do all you are doing." What if I left my wife and family? What if I fail as a caregiver? I am expected by family and peers to succeed. If I fail, will I then be ostracized by my family and ridiculed by my peers?

After much reflection and soul searching, I have come to the conclusion that I must continue doing my best and then let the chips fall where they may. It's easy for my wife's family to have high expectations of me; it's easy for people to tell me what I should be doing as a caregiver. It is easy for other family members to say, "Glenn, why aren't you doing this?" Or, "Why haven't you done that?" They don't live in my house. They don't know the pressures I have to deal with. Tending to the needs of a chronically ill patient three-hundred-sixty-five days a year, is vastly different than spending the weekend.

No one can know what being a caregiver is like until they've done it. People often visualize themselves caring for a parent or spouse. They think to themselves, "This is what I would do." They may even come to you and explain exactly what you're doing wrong and how to correct the situation. They sincerely believe this is helpful. The only fly in the ointment is they don't have the slightest idea of what they're talking about.

I'm not sure there is any way to put a good spin on this subject. None of us can fully live up to somebody else's expectations. I don't think I could ever do all that my wife's family thinks I should. I'm trying. That's all I can do.

Many times you will be asked how the patient is doing. Seldom will you be asked how you are doing. The average person doesn't think about it. After all you're not the one who is sick.

The last thing people want or expect to hear from you is complaining. Their expectation is that you are committed to the task of caregiver and therefore, why should you complain. They consider it to be your lot in life--that's just the way things are. If you want to run all your friends off then spend all your time complaining about how bad everything is.

I think in my role as a minister that people like to see me smile and say everything is wonderful. When people ask me on Sunday morning, "I see your wife is not with you today. Is she feeling worse?" Normally I will say she is doing fine. When the question is pressed a little farther, "Why didn't she come?" Then it is difficult to avoid a clear-cut answer. A truthful answer in no way matches the expectation of the person asking the question. "Well she didn't come to church this morning because her hands were so numb that she couldn't button her dress. And since her hands are so numb she knew people like you would insist on shaking hands with her." Another truthful answer, "She was almost out the door when her bladder gave way and she soaked her dress. We could have changed her and brought her on, but after you have spent two hours getting dressed and soak yourself with urine just as you're going out the door, well it tends to take the fun out of it."

When you tell people the truth it puts them in the position of having to react. This makes some people very uncomfortable. They don't expect you to lie to them, nor do they expect hard, unvarnished honesty.

I think the best way to sum up this chapter is to say that care giving is a constant struggle between good and best. You know you have chosen to do the right thing by caring for your son, daughter, mother, father, husband or wife. You are doing your best to live up to everyone's expectations of what is good enough for the patient. But somehow, no matter how hard you try or how diligent you are you feel you have fallen far short of everyone's expectations. Take heart, you are the one who has to live with yourself and stand before God. The Lord is merciful and forgiving. He will never expect perfection, only that you try and do your best.

Chapter 21

Down They Go and Everybody Else with Them

By nature I am a very positive upbeat person. But if I am going to be honest and realistic, I must tell you that when someone you love suffers, you suffer right along with the individual.

I have seen Karen struggle and weep. I have struggled and wept with her. She has been in the depths of despair. I have been in the depths of despair with her. You can't love someone and care for them and stand idly by and watch them battle extreme physical and emotional pain without paying a toll. Sometimes the price is tremendous.

When we continually dwell on the negative aspects of life our attitude and disposition can become one of depression. There are three factors that weigh heavily in the development of depression: injustice, anger and indecision.

Karen has asked the question as many people do, when confronted with a serious illness, why me? Everyone who is sick or injured goes through the "why me" stage. She hates not being the strong healthy woman she once was. She has railed against God and everybody else it seems at the

137

injustice she has suffered. Many times spoken through anger and tears she has expressed how unfair life has been to her.

I, too, feel it is unfair. I don't think anyone should have to suffer through such an awful debilitating disease as multiple sclerosis. But life isn't fair. There are millions of people who suffer from multiple sclerosis, muscular dystrophy, blindness, one leg, one arm, stroke victims, terminal cancer, and accident victims ad infinitum.

I would love to have Karen back as the vibrant wonderful woman that she was the first ten years of our marriage, that's only human. And it's only human to feel unfairly burdened with all the responsibilities that weigh heavily on my shoulders; coupled with Karen's declining health I could quite easily become depressed and discouraged. I could wallow in self-pity about my lot in life as a caregiver, or I can choose to channel that negative energy elsewhere: a firm and abiding trust in God, my children, exercise, work and writing.

When we nurse anger about our situation in life and harbor ill will against those we love or even against ourselves, it eats away at the very core of our being. We become prime candidates for depression.

The caregiver may harbor angry feelings about all that is expected of him. You may be caring for a patient who is struggling with his or her own issues of anger and resentment. In this situation the patient has few outlets to vent these negative emotions; hence you as the caregiver take the brunt of their anger. The anger of the care receiver can then easily feed the anger of the caregiver.

People have carried the burden of anger, hate and resentment in their heart for years. Have you ever known an angry person who was happy? I dare say the answer is no. Chronic unhappiness leads to chronic depression and that is a most unhealthy situation.

Indecision is another cause of depression. This may seem like an inappropriate term, but it is not. You will be faced with countless decisions. Ideally you will make these decisions in conjunction with the patient, however the time will come when your loved one is no longer able to express his or her wishes. You must face these decisions on your own. This can be a great source of pressure.

You can spend weeks and months trying to decide on the correct course of action. You want to do the right thing. You pray and consider all the options and then you must make a decision. If you continue to vacillate it will only lead to frustration and depression. Therefore, you make the best-informed decision possible and proceed forward.

Chapter 22

What About Guilt?

Care giving is something we do because the bottom line is we love the patient and care about their welfare. We feel responsible. We feel committed. We want to do the right thing.

Most caregivers feel as though they live their lives on an emotional roller coaster. Going for years hoping things will get better. Feeling bitter and discouraged when we see our loved one steadily declining before our eyes. Believing that each new medication will be the one to turn everything around, and then being disappointed. We strive to do everything possible for the patient. But sometimes our best just isn't good enough. There are days when we feel as though we've hit a brick wall and have failed miserably.

Guilt enters the picture when we are physically and mentally exhausted, when we're just plain tired of doing the right thing. When we are rested and focused, then we can cope with the pressures that we face. But when I've had a short night of sleep and a long day of activity, it's much harder to plaster a smile on my face when I'm struggling to lift Karen into the car, or when I've just issued the last and final wake-up call to the boys. You may be a rock. But even the biggest and strongest rock may begin to crumble around the edges.

The son or daughter who has spent years caring for an ailing mother feels guilty when there is no choice left except to take mother to a nursing home. We feel guilty every time we walk out the door and leave our loved one alone. I struggled with guilt writing this book.

In my quest for honesty, I've divulged some very personal and sensitive information about my family and myself. I have thought, "No, I am not going to write this book." And then a week would pass and once again I am struck by the realization of just how little material is available for caregivers.

There are twenty million Americans that are individually or collectively responsible for the care of a parent, spouse or child. Finding a support group for caregivers has been like looking for a needle in a haystack. It would have meant so much to me if I could have found a group of caregivers to share my feelings and emotions with. To affirm, if you will, that I am not alone in my struggle.

So, despite my initial reservations, I will continue forward with this book in the hopes that by doing so I can help others who find themselves in the same predicament.

Multiple sclerosis has changed our lives. Karen's disease has robbed her of her health and the ability to enjoy many of life's simplest pleasures. As her husband and caregiver I feel robbed too. Yes, I feel I am missing out on life. That was a difficult statement to make. I am a very private person. It isn't easy for me to admit that I feel cheated and at times resentful, because my wife is sick. It makes me feel lousy. It makes feel selfish. It makes me feel guilty.

There have been many days when I listened to Karen express her feelings of isolation and bitterness towards her situation and MS. And I have thought, "Do you think this is easy on me?" Then I feel extremely guilty for having such a thought.

The fact that you are locked into caring for someone is in every way a very confining situation. You have to stay in touch throughout the day. Planning an overnight business trip becomes a major ordeal. You feel trapped, and you don't like it. You feel guilty for having these feelings.

It's only natural to feel as though you're missing out on some of life's pleasures, because you are. It's only natural to feel confined by your duties as a caregiver, because you are. It's natural to feel some resentment because of the difficulties you are experiencing. Be honest with yourself. Don't pretend you love being a caregiver. It alleviates a lot of pressure and stress when you can openly admit to yourself that you hate it. Don't pretend that everything is wonderful, you're not fooling anyone, least of all yourself. Once you have said to your inner circle of friends, "I don't like being a caregiver," then you are free to be yourself.

Everybody needs help. Don't feel guilty about seeking comfort and guidance. A good counselor will be invaluable to you in your journey as a caregiver. I personally feel a good counselor is someone who has a personal walk with God. Such a person uses the resources of psychological training combined with an understanding of God's Word.

You didn't feel guilty about wanting to retire, did you? You didn't feel guilty about looking forward to your child graduating from college, did you? You didn't feel guilty about wanting to get away from a condescending demanding boss, did you? Then don't feel guilty because you want to escape the pain and frustrations of being a caregiver. Stop being so hard on yourself. You're only human and you're doing the best you can.

You don't have to feel guilty. Put your situation in God's hands. God never intended us to live a life of guilt. He gave His Son Jesus Christ to die on the cross for our sins. You will never feel as though you've been a perfect caregiver. You must say, "I am doing the best I can."

Chapter 23

Trust and Its Impact on Relationships

Trust is vital in any relationship. Where there is no trust there is no pure communication or revelation of the self.

Trust between the caregiver and the care receiver is one of the most dynamic aspects of the relationship. The patient should have the assurance that the caregiver, whether a parent, spouse or child, will be there.

As a husband for over twenty-four years and a minister, my wife has confidence in me. She trusts that I will keep a roof over her head and food on the table. She is confident that she will always have a safe, warm place to sleep and clothes to wear; this is how it ought to be in our world. Spouses should be able to depend on each other. Parents and children and brothers and sisters and Christian people in general should have a spirit and a heart that goes out to others in their time of need.

This kind of trust and confidence is good and bad. Being able to believe in somebody is one of the greatest feelings in the world. But trust and confidence can also be abused. For example, the Christian has confidence that he may completely trust in God's love demonstrated in His Son Christ. God knows every flaw and imperfection and loves us still. This is a wonderful feeling. We sin and fall short over and over yet we still have confidence that we are loved and forgiven. However, the confidence we have experienced from His mercy, should never be taken as a license to steal, lie and kill. Nor does the trust we have in the Lord mean we can live life to the extreme without paying the penalty. "God, I know you love me and are going to take care of me; therefore, I am going to drive one hundred miles an hour on a country road." Or, "God, I know you want the best for me, so I'm going to smoke three packs of cigarettes a day and believe that you, God, will keep me from having lung cancer." Or, "God, I'm just going to sit on the couch and eat pizza and trust you to keep me from being overweight."

We reap what we sow. This principal relates to every aspect of our lives. There are limitations on how far we can push and try God; and, there are limitations on how far we can push and try people.

My father worked in a coal mine for over thirty years to raise five kids and take care of a wife. He provided for me and made it financially possible for me to go to college. I give him high marks for that.

Dad tolerated a lot of the usual nonsense from me when I was a teenager. He loved me, but there were limits. I knew as a boy how far I could push the boundary line.

When I was fifteen years old my first cousin Kevin and I were left alone at my parent's house. Mom and Dad had gone to church. My parents had only been gone about twenty minutes when I got the bright idea of taking Dad's truck for a drive. Kevin, who was a year older than I, immediately agreed. I found my dad's spare key and in no time we were driving down Milo road.

We drove on for about twenty minutes before heading to the neighboring community of Richardson. We ended up on a dark, winding, gravel road. You probably have a good idea where this story is leading. We took one of the turns a little too fast and ended up at the bottom of a steep embankment. Directly across the road was a little country church. There was a huge revival meeting going on with two hundred or more people in attendance. It seemed like every one of them funneled out the church doors down to where Kevin and I were climbing out of the truck. It was awful.

We walked down the road to a house where a man and his wife allowed us to use their telephone to call a wrecker service and my uncle. The wrecker pulled the truck out of the ditch and Kevin rode home with his father. In the mean time, I drove the crippled truck home.

My Dad was standing in the doorway of the front porch, waiting for me. I knew I had done wrong and made a dreadful decision, and what's more, I was terrified as any fifteen year old boy would be under the circumstances. I was convinced he would kill me and ask questions later.

We had a little building out behind our house with a gas heater and a bed. My dad used to sleep there during the day when he worked third shift. I parked the truck and made a beeline for that little building. I wanted to avoid my dad at all costs.

Within a minute he was out the door. "Glenn are you all right?"

"Yes," I replied.

"Get in the house," he ordered.

I didn't know what to expect. I was too big for a whipping, I hoped. I already felt miserable and stupid for taking the truck. A tongue lashing from my dad at that point would have been worse than any belt or spanking.

"Glenn, don't ever say anything to me about a driver's license. I don't even want to hear about that."

That was the end of the discussion. Well, I did get my driver's license a few months later when I turned sixteen, but I always wondered after that whether or not my father trusted me.

The child believes mom and dad will be there for them. Mom and Dad believe the child will help them in times of crisis. The care receiver who has been married for a number of years believes the spouse will see them through their illness. Surely this is the way it should be.

This trust and confidence in the caregiver should not be perverted into a false sense of security. The point I want to make is that trust does not give one the right to be abusive. The patient does not have the right to verbally assault the caregiver. Unfortunately, in many cases they do.

A lady confided to me about her father who had passed away from cancer. Her father was bedfast for a number of months before his death, during which time his wife had cared for him in their home. "There was nothing my mother could do to please him. He was verbally abusive to mother and everyone in the family. He didn't have a good word to say. His trust level that we would continue to care for him was incredible."

A young girl that graduated from the same high school I did died from multiple sclerosis. A friend of mine went to visit her about a year before her death. The friend reported, "We went to see her but we never went back. She was bitter and rude and she was so ugly about her condition that we didn't have the heart to go back."

It is normal for us to shy away from people who are in a bad mood. Unpleasant people are not attractive. Unpleasant circumstances repel us. The fact that you are feeling stressed and weary by a care receiver who starts berating you the minute you walk through the door is a natural reaction to a bad situation.

The patient may feel they are in a protective zone because of their illness. They also feel confident that you are always going to be there to care for them no matter how difficult or abusive they may become.

Sickness does not give anyone a license to stretch the confidence and trust level of the caregiver to the ultimate limit.

Try talking to the patient. Explain to them that even though they are sick, they do not have the right to berate those who are trying to help them. This may cause the care receiver to stop and think about their behavior, or it may get you nowhere.

One lonely night when Karen was in the throes of an especially violent reaction to prednisone I called a neurologist. I told him my wife was killing the entire family and me. He didn't have an immediate answer for me, but after some thought recommended she see a counselor. All the counseling in the world wouldn't have had any effect on what the prednisone was doing to her nervous system. What she really needed was an anti-depressant to help control the violent mood swings that were practically destroying our family.

The neurologist offered me very little practical help, and I'm sorry to say that has too often been the case. Don't expect a lot of help from your doctor. I wish I didn't have to share that with you, but it's a fact you need to learn quickly. You must do all you can to educate yourself about your loved one's disease and the medications they are prescribed. Don't rely on a doctor who sees hundreds of patients a month to take a personal interest in your case.

There is a limit to the verbal pounding. We are only human, and as such, we have our breaking points. You may need to lay your cards on the table. Tell the patient, "I love you and care about you. I want to do everything I can to help you, but if you don't stop talking to me and the family in this hateful, unkind way, I'll load you in the car and take you to the first nursing home I can find."

You may have to fulfill this threat for your sake and the sake of everyone in the household.

You may legitimately wonder, does this person not appreciate all I do for them? You may feel as though they are demanding your services because they trust you never to desert them. You must look within for strength and put yourself in God's hands. We cannot survive this journey alone.

Chapter 24

Medical Costs

Multiple sclerosis or any chronic illness, which requires on going medical care and supervision, is going to be an expensive proposition. Given the choice, we would all rather spend our hard-earned cash on a dinner out with the family. However, when illness strikes, do we question the cost? I think not. When you're sick and need surgery, you don't complain about the fee for the operating room. When I witnessed the birth of my sons, I didn't care about the hospital bill. When my father had cancer surgery to remove part of his colon, cost was the least of my concerns.

In the ten plus years since Karen was diagnosed with MS, I have become increasingly disillusioned with the health care industry. I think the word "industry" perhaps says it all. We are effectively dehumanizing ourselves to mere numbers and case files. Hospital stays and medical procedures are now dependent on what our HMO or insurance company is willing to subsidize. The patient has been forgotten in the quest for profits.

The effects of long term medical care for the average middle to upper middle class family in America can be devastating. The months turn into years; the medical bills slowly and steadily mount, gnawing away at the family's savings. This is why many people lose their homes when faced with a health-related crisis. Many families have no alternative but to file for bankruptcy. A case in point, a man came to me for counseling who had been struggling for a number of years with medical bills. "I have to file bankruptcy. I have a family to take care of. I have a ton of medical bills. I've looked at every alternative. I can't get any more money on my house. What choice do I have?"

What choice indeed. The family who has someone in the home with a chronic illness, who is dependent on medical treatment for their very survival, has no choice. In one year our current hospitalization premium has increased twenty percent. We are in a do or die situation. We can't really afford the high premiums--and yet we can't afford not to pay them.

When Karen took medical leave from her teaching position, she eventually qualified for disabled social security benefits. Social Security amounts to a fraction of what her original salary was, but let me hasten to say we are grateful for this monthly income. When Karen qualified for social security benefits, she received a Medicare medical card. Medicare part A covers hospital stays and all services rendered to the patient while in the hospital. Medicare does not pay for prescription drugs.

When Karen was on a regimen of Beta Seron, prednizone, anti-depressants, and muscle relaxants, our monthly pharmaceutical bill ranged from $1200.00 to $1500.00 per month. Who in America--unless you are independently wealthy--can afford that kind of expense on top of all your other monthly obligations?

It became imperative to our financial survival to maintain Karen's insurance policy that was part of her benefits package while still teaching school in Kentucky. In order to do this, we had to maintain our residence in Kentucky. As a result, we paid state taxes in Kentucky and Indiana. Why not switch insurance companies, you may ask. The answer is simple. Insurance companies do not want to insure people who have a chronic illness. Most insurance companies will not cover a pre-existing condition such as MS, heart disease, or cancer. Our insurance was also tied to a plan where the insured had to be a resident of the state.

Karen's insurance policy pays 80% of the cost for prescription drugs, which still leaves the patient responsible for the remaining 20%. Our average monthly expenditure for medication is usually at or about three hundred dollars. Three hundred dollars is a huge chunk of our budget. Can you imagine what people do who aren't fortunate enough to have insurance coverage? They simply go without the medical care they need. That's the hard, cold reality of the situation.

When Karen was confined to a wheelchair I learned about the Home Health Care industry. Home Health Care groups have sprung up around America like the dandelions spring up in my front yard during the springtime. I couldn't believe how quickly the representative was in my house with her legs under my kitchen table getting the necessary information for Karen's application. She was pleasant and genuinely seemed sympathetic to our situation. What wonderful people, I thought. What a wonderful occupation. These people have a special calling in life.

There are many things I could say about the Home Health Care industry. For one, they are opportunists who prey upon vulnerable people who are sick and frightened and in desperate need of help. Secondly, the inflated figures they submitted to Medicare for services rendered were little better than fraud.

For one month, Home Health Care submitted a bill to Medicare for $4300.00. In one year, just for Karen alone, Home Health Care would collect $50,000.00 from Medicare. Let's break this down item by item. Home Health Care billed Medicare $100.00 for each visit to our home. These visits were for a one-hour duration. The Home Health Care aid, who by the way was not a nurse, helped Karen bathe and then dress. Another $1300.00 was billed to Medicare for a registered nurse and a physical therapist who came once a week.

Every representative we spoke to from the Home Health Care groups told us that Medicare would only pay 80% of the billed fee. They assured us that we would not be responsible for the remaining 20%, that the 80% fee collected from Medicare would be sufficient for their company. I can imagine it would be.

As of March 1998, our Home Health Care supplier told us they would no longer be able to help us. New guidelines and restrictions by Medicare had been established. Karen would now be limited to $4000.00 per year of coverage from Medicare for the type of care she required.

This has been a real hardship for our family. At the present time we are looking for someone to take over the duties of the Home Health Care aid; but finding an honest, dependable person who will work for what I can afford to pay is not an easy assignment.

For the present I have taken over the task of bathing and dressing Karen and getting her ready to face the day. Right now all that is required is my time. I am fortunate as a pastor that my church doesn't say I must be at my office at 7:00 a.m. My working hours are more flexible than most people's by the shear nature of the work I do. Many caregivers are not as lucky. Their work schedule is non-negotiable.

This is why some people have no choice except to have their loved one placed in a nursing home or long-term care facility. Long-term care is very expensive and Medicare does not cover the cost. There is a government-sponsored program, Medicaid, which provides assistance to the poverty stricken.

On the surface Medicaid sounds like the answer to many of our prayers, but it is not. In order to qualify you must prove you are financially without means. A married couple with one spouse working will not qualify. However, if the working spouse divorces the invalid leaving them with nothing, the long-term care facility will confiscate what little assets are left from the patient and then Medicaid will take over the cost of the nursing home.

This is not uncommon, I'm sad to say. One couple who attends my church has never legally married because it would have affected her Medicaid status and would have cut out her medical and financial supplements. Financially it would have been devastating for this couple.

I can't judge these people, I would never presume to do such a thing. I believe wholeheartedly that we must do what is legally and morally right. Is it morally right for a nation to penalize a couple who is legally married? Is it right that couples who live together but who are not considered legally married in the eyes of the state be compensated? It is a cruel system that values the dollar more highly than human dignity.

These questions will have to be addressed by you and I, our lawmakers and insurance providers, and the citizens of our country. I know that as a caregiver you are stressed some days to your limit. You don't think you have the stamina and emotional fortitude to go out and promote changes in our government. If I can find time to write this book, then I must find a few minutes to call my congressman and write letters to those government representatives who can make a difference and help right this national wrong. We must all make the time! We are the only ones who have a heart felt understanding of this personal and national crisis.

In conclusion let me say that I know how devastating financial worries can be. There have been times when all I wanted to do was crawl under the bed and just cry the day away. But that kind of worry and anxiety isn't going to make the medical bills go away.

159

Be concerned. There is a difference between worry and concern. You are concerned or you wouldn't be reading this chapter. Keep in mind that the situation you find yourself in is only temporary. It may last a long time but nothing in this life is permanent. The financial woes you have from medical costs and your care giving responsibilities are not forever.

People in America must go back to helping each other. We have become a society of people who live behind closed doors. We push a button and the garage door opens; we push another button and the door closes isolating us from the world. We need one another in our society. We need to help one another and we need to trust in God.

Chapter 25

Housing Becomes a Major Issue

I think one of the most difficult issues that you face as a caregiver is housing. Whether you are caring for a spouse, elderly parent, or perhaps you are thinking about your senior years; your home should be a place of comfort and refuge.

When a person is confined to a wheelchair, steps become a major concern. In 1993 we moved to a large two-story house in Louisa, Kentucky. Karen at the time was still walking. We had continued to hope that her MS was not chronic progressive and that a remission was just around the corner. Sadly, that remission was never forth coming.

As the disease progressed, it became increasingly difficult for Karen to manage the stairs to the second story of the house where the boys' bedrooms were. It was a chore for her to drag her leg up the steps. Soon it was no longer a chore to go up the steps; it was impossible. By the time we were ready to move out of the house Karen had completely stopped going upstairs.

I had spent years dreaming about living in a big house. When I got into my big house I spent over two years trying to get out of it. Happiness is not found in big houses. Happiness is never found in possessions.

When we finally sold the two-story house we knew we had to find something that was self-contained on one level. I also wanted a house that would be in close proximity to my church. This narrowed our search down considerably. We finally found a house that met all our criteria. It was a new home about half the size of the Louisa house. It is very functional, easy to heat and cool. We have three bedrooms, a small living room, dining room, family room, and 2 ½ baths, along with a large covered back porch and two-car garage.

Our smaller house has been a real blessing for Karen. She can travel in her wheelchair from one end of the house to the other very quickly. She can call out to the boys or I if she needs anything and there is never a problem hearing her or getting to her quickly.

Please don't misunderstand if I seem to be singing the praises of a smaller house compared to a larger house. But as a caregiver of a wife who is in a wheelchair I was forced to take a good hard look at the advantages of smaller one level houses. Smaller houses certainly require less maintenance; utility bills for fuel and electricity will be considerably lower and less space means less house cleaning.

A self-contained home on one level is advantageous if you are caring for an elderly person. A friend of mine brought his mother from out of state to live with him and his wife. He felt his house was unsuitable for his mother because of the stairs. He soon found a one level house well suited to his needs.

Let me take this opportunity to expound a bit, if I may, about caring for one's aging parents. Bringing a parent into your home requires a lifestyle change. You and your mother or father, whatever the case may be, haven't lived together for perhaps twenty or thirty years. There has been a radical role reversal; you are now in the position of caring for them. By the shear nature of the situation tension and misunderstandings can arise.

When another person is suddenly added to the household everyone tends to feel a bit claustrophobic. Whatever you can do to ensure the privacy of your family will certainly help ease the tension and make for an easier transition.

One couple I know had to bring the man's mother into their home to live. He was fortunate to be able to remodel a wing of his house to provide a small apartment for his mother. This worked out well. The mother still had a place where she could close the door and have her privacy.

As much as I love my parents I know that living with them every day would be much more difficult than a weekend visit. As the old cliché goes, "familiarity breeds contempt." When we haven't lived in the same house with someone for a number of years, we tend to forget the petty little annoyances that drove us to distraction. Living with people, seeing them each morning at the breakfast table and saying goodnight day in and day out can have its trying moments.

Let's be realistic, shall we. Houses are expensive items. Not everyone can afford to remodel their existing home for an aging parent, and not everyone can afford to buy a larger one level house to accommodate an extra person. Be creative. Do whatever is within your means to provide as much privacy as possible for all concerned.

Buying a house with all of life's stages in mind is a wise investment. You may regret that large two-story house with the laundry room in the basement when you approach your senior years. Just a word to the wise if you are considering purchasing or building a new house.

A one level house with easy access is the best-case scenario for your loved one. This is something by the way that not only benefits the patient, but the day and time may come when you too will appreciate your purchase.

Chapter 26

Traveling with the Patient

I love to travel. I love the spontaneity of jumping into the car and heading out. I love the freedom of boarding a plane and flying across the country.

In this day and age our travel options seem unlimited. We can choose to journey by automobile, train, airplane, bus, and even cruise ship if the fancy takes us--that is, if you have two strong legs. Multiple sclerosis has changed all that.

Traveling with an invalid is a major hurdle. It is by no means an impossible hurdle to overcome but you must plan your agenda before stepping one foot outside your front door. The old saying, "If you fail to plan, you are planning to fail," rings very true when traveling with someone who is confined to a wheelchair.

For example, the last long car trip Karen and our family took together was from Newburgh, Indiana to New Orleans. At that time Karen was still able to transfer from the wheelchair without our assistance. When the family needed to stop we could help Karen into the wheelchair and she could use the facilities at the interstate rest areas.

As time and the disease progressed, Karen needed more and more help to transfer from the wheelchair to the commode. Stopping at a roadside rest area became impossible.

Karen's family lives in Dayton, Ohio, which is a five-hour drive from Newburgh. Does this mean she never again goes to visit her family in Dayton? In our situation the answer to that question is no.

Making a five-hour trip requires thought and planning. Five hours is simply too long to be cooped up in a car without a restroom break. I can't do it, my children can't do it, so how can I expect my wife to do it?

In our case, the halfway point between Newburgh and Dayton is Louisville, Kentucky. The staff at the Holiday Inn on Zorn Avenue in Louisville has always been very congenial and accommodating. When we arrive at the Inn, I help Karen into the wheelchair and wheel her into the hotel lobby. I ask the desk clerk if I may wheel my wife into the ladies restroom. After obtaining permission the desk clerk will usually stand outside the restroom door while I help Karen. On occasion one of the boys will stand guard to explain my presence in the ladies room should anyone need to use the facilities while I am with my wife. The need for someone outside the restroom door is a must. I have always feared some unsuspecting woman would walk into the ladies room and be startled by my presence.

Since we are discussing automobile travel at this juncture, let me emphasize the importance of driving a dependable vehicle.

We drove one of our cars to New Orleans and had a great trip. The journey was smooth and uneventful. When we returned to Southern Indiana, we decided to make a quick trip to Kentucky to visit my family. On the way back to Indiana from Kentucky the engine began making a very disturbing noise. By the time we made it to the exit for the Holiday Inn, I feared we were in for some real problems. I can't tell you how thankful I was to park the car and wheel Karen into the cool hotel lobby. Pushing a wheelchair along the interstate on a hot day in June is a very grim prospect.

The hotel staff was most helpful. They supplied me with names and numbers of garages and towing services and offered their lobby as a resting place for Karen and the boys while I tried to sort out our dilemma. And sort it out, I did, but not without a great deal of difficulty and more than a little stress.

Just imagine how disastrous our situation would have been if we had been stranded along a deserted stretch of highway or if we had been traveling at night.

Since that incident, when we travel I have made it a point to rent a car. You can arrange for an unlimited mileage rate and a weeklong rental for less than a single month's car payment. The expense of the rental is well worth the peace of mind it gives to our family and me.

When traveling any distance make sure you have a credit card for unexpected problems—breakdowns, extra cash, or what have you. Another invaluable aid to traveling with a handicapped person is the cellular phone. Remember you are traveling with someone who could experience a medical emergency at any time. With a cellular phone at your disposal you can dial 911 and have an ambulance and medical help dispatched to your location. Peace of mind and knowing that you have prepared for a medical emergency is well worth the monthly expenditure.

Traveling also entails lodging. It is amazing how small many hotel rooms are and how few hotels have rooms that are accessible for the handicapped. The doorways leading into the room and bathroom must be wide enough to allow a wheelchair easy access. We have stayed at hotels where there was not enough space in the bathroom for Karen to wheel herself in and transfer to the commode. In that situation, I literally had to lift Karen out of her chair, drag her across the bathroom, and help her onto the toilet seat. After a few such experiences we began consulting a travel agent before starting out on a trip. A travel agent can help you book accommodations that you know beforehand will be suitable for someone in the patient's condition.

Perhaps you are thinking to yourself, why not fly and cut the travel time in half? Wouldn't that be an easier alternative for the patient? Unfortunately the answer is no. Boarding a plane for someone in a wheelchair is a major undertaking. Can you imagine having a special lift pick you up and load you on the plane like a piece of luggage while fifty or more other passengers look on? Then after you are finally aboard, you must try to navigate to an assigned seat. The small planes that fly in and out of our regional airport have very narrow aisles. Making Karen comfortable in that situation would be impossible. More important even than physical comfort would be the loss of dignity she would suffer.

You've finally made it to your destination. Plan on a relatively short visit. Bear in mind that if you are staying with friends or family that most people do not live in homes that are suited to the needs of the handicapped. A stay of one or two nights is manageable. A prolonged visit puts a strain not only on your hosts, but on the patient as well.

In conclusion, let me assure you that traveling with a handicapped person is possible but difficult, and at times very frustrating. With all the work and planning involved you may be tempted to throw up your hands in despair and say, "Forget it!" But you mustn't. You can still travel as a family. You can still visit old friends and unfamiliar places. Granted, the journey will be a little different, but well worth it.

Chapter 27

Shopping for my Wife

Regardless of who it is, it is never easy to shop for someone else. Try to imagine being stuck at home and sending your spouse, child or parent on an errand to the mall for the basic necessities of life. I can't imagine anyone shopping for me to my complete satisfaction.

Put yourself in the patient's position. You have spent time and energy compiling a shopping list. Among the items on your list are coffee, toothpaste and black socks. Sounds simple enough, but when the caregiver presents the items, the care receiver discovers to their dismay that the coffee is not the brand they enjoy, the socks are wool instead of cotton, and the toothpaste contains baking soda instead of fluoride.

The patient is frustrated because what they consider a simple request has not been met. The caregiver is frustrated because he took time out of his busy day to make a trip to an overcrowded mall, search for each one of the items, and now he feels unappreciated because the patient is upset and angry about his selections.

As a caregiver and care receiver you certainly have enough obstacles to overcome without hassling over shopping mishaps. But lets face it--it's distressing.

During the years that Karen was healthy she did the grocery shopping. It was something she wanted to do. She enjoyed it. As Karen became more disabled, I took over this responsibility. It wouldn't have been such a problem for me had I not been expected to purchase some very personal items for my wife. We develop so many little hang-ups in our society. Looking for and purchasing bladder pads was my hang-up.

When I first started shopping for Karen, I had no idea where the bladder pads were located in the store or even what brand name to purchase. It took a considerable amount of time and courage on my part to work up the nerve to ask a clerk to help me locate bladder pads. I just knew they would look at me funny, because I felt so terribly conspicuous about the request.

Now why should I feel self-conscious about the items I purchase in a grocery store? In the beginning I suppose, I feared what other people might think.

I had a very unfortunate incident when I first began shopping for Karen. I was feeling edgy and self-conscious when I walked into the store; I dreaded the thought of walking up to the counter carrying nothing but a huge box of bladder pads. I went so far as to get a shopping cart, filling it with a few items that we really didn't need just to avoid standing in line with those pads in my arms. When my turn at the checkout came I placed the items on the conveyor belt, waiting nervously for the clerk to ring up my purchases. The clerk was a young man in his early twenties. Obviously, he was inexperienced and immature. Taking the box of pads in his hand he said, "Well, I'm not going to ask about these." I wasn't going to justify his rudeness with a reply. I paid for the items and walked out of the store.

That clerk and his unprofessional remarks were the reason for my insecurity. Who wants to be confronted at the checkout line in the presence of other customers about what you have or have not placed in your cart?

I want to hasten to add that I have moved beyond that paranoia. I can look back on that incident with a certain amount of humor. Now when I go to the checkout I just toss those things up on the counter like I would a loaf of bread. I mean after all--who really cares.

Another hurdle I had to overcome was the ladies lingerie and hosiery department. Going into a major department store shopping for thigh-high stockings has been quite an experience. To start, I feel like a fish out of water

173

among all those women as I finger through racks and racks of packaged stockings. Nine times out of ten I can't find the size and color Karen requested. You may be wondering, "Why don't you just go ask a clerk?" Have you ever tried wading through a bunch of women standing in line to pay for stockings on a Saturday morning? It's impossible. Plus I feel very conspicuous just being in the lingerie department. I have learned to swallow my pride, get in line and wait my turn to ask the clerk for help. Of course it takes her less than a minute to locate the correct size and color. Slowly, I am learning the ropes in the hosiery department. It is still not something I enjoy doing, but as with everything else, repetition does bring results.

Another challenge I have met, but I can't confess to having mastered it completely, is the cosmetic department. Karen sends me to the store with a slip of paper specifying the color and brand name of the cosmetics she needs. I have learned in this process that there are different bottles and tubes that claim to do everything. The help of a clerk is always essential.

My greatest difficulty has been getting the right product. This often happens because the clerk sees me coming, rather like a dishonest auto mechanic will see a trusting, but uninformed customer coming with a car in need of repairs. When I get home Karen quickly points out my error and sends me back in quick fashion to make the exchange.

I am slightly more at ease in the cosmetic department, because you are likely to find more men milling about. I don't feel so lonely.

I have found several of the ladies from our church have been most helpful about running errands for Karen. This will take a considerable load off your shoulders if you can occasionally call upon a woman friend or volunteer to buy these personal items for your loved one. This of course holds true if you are a woman caregiver faced with shopping for your husband.

Let me say in conclusion that this can become a very sensitive issue. More than one heated argument has occurred because of a mistaken purchase. Your attitude as the caregiver should be one of understanding. I know it isn't always easy to be understanding when you are on your way back to an overcrowded mall to exchange lipstick and eyeliner, but do your best. I have tried to develop the happy-go-lucky attitude that this is just another little part of the journey.

Chapter 28

You Better Have a Sense of Humor

People in our society need humor. We need to be able to laugh and cast our cares aside. Comedy clubs have sprung up all over America. There is now a cable channel devoted solely to comedy. People stay up late to watch Jay Leno and David Letterman.

Humor is a wonderful outlet for the stress we encounter in the daily grind of work, family and responsibilities. My father worked long hard hours in a coal mine most of his adult life. My dad has a great sense of humor. There were days as a child when I remember him coming home from the mines tired and cranky. But I also remember that my father loved to laugh. Thirty years slaving away in a coal mine takes its toll, but his sense of humor and the ability to look on the lighter side was a great escape for him. Is it any wonder then, that the caregiver who daily encounters depression and illness finds humor an invaluable asset in relieving stress and anxiety?

I had lived in Newburgh only a short time when I met a gentleman whose wife had been diagnosed with MS. The disease had progressed to the point that she became totally dependent upon a wheelchair. Fortunately, in this woman's case the disease went into remission and today she appears to be like every other normal healthy woman her age.

One day when we were having coffee, this gentleman confided to me, "You better develop a sense of humor." This was excellent advice, and now I want to pass it along to you. If you don't learn to laugh, you'll surely learn to cry.

With all the stress and tension that comes with caring for someone who is chronically ill, the caregiver can become so bogged down with the daily routine of life there's scarcely time to sit down and read a funny book or enjoy a movie.

We rent a movie almost every week. I am very careful in my selection. Caregivers should make it a point to watch lighthearted films and avoid movies that are intense or have sad themes. Often Karen watches these movies with the boys and I. It's good for her to be able to lose herself for a brief time and laugh along with us.

As I've stated before exercise has a very therapeutic effect upon me. When I go to the gym for an intense workout, my mood always improves as endorphins are released into my bloodstream. Half way through an aerobics class I have been known to chuckle and on occasion to break out laughing.

Sometimes I chuckle taking care of Karen. I laugh at myself when I'm trying to put on her underwear and I goof up. Or, I'm putting on her stockings and make a complete mess of it. There have been times when I have been overcome with laughter at my mistakes. Please understand I am not talking about sarcastic humor. I am talking about the ability to find the humor in a situation. I have never laughed at Karen. I have cried with her, but never laughed at her.

Don't let illness and worry steal your joy. There is a difference between having a good laugh and joy. Humor is external. Joy is internal. We can laugh our brains out and be crying on the inside.

The Bible speaks of joy. "The fruit of the spirit is joy," (Galatians 5:22). Joy is deep and abiding. Joy is ongoing. When you have a bad day the quiet presence of joy will see you through the chaos of life. Internal joy enables you to laugh with peace of mind.

I don't want to leave the impression that I laugh about my wife's disease or what it has done to my family. I take that very seriously. However, developing an attitude that finds the humor in all that we have to go through seems to make some of the moments a little lighter.

Chapter 29

Going Out to Eat

Going out to eat under the best of circumstances can be a lesson or a trial in patience. Escorting someone in a wheelchair into a crowded restaurant lobby can be an even greater trial.

Our family has always enjoyed going out to a restaurant for lunch or dinner. Since Karen's illness has progressed we do not go out now as often as we once did. When Karen was teaching and I was working on several projects at once, it was much easier for us to go to a restaurant than to take the time and energy necessary to prepare a meal at home.

We have had many good experiences at restaurants and some that weren't so good. When I use the phrase "good experience," I'm not referring to the quality of our food, but to the accessibility of the establishment and the overall cooperation of the staff.

Wheeling Karen into a crowded restaurant is always a little tricky. A large number of people milling about a relatively small room makes maneuvering her wheelchair more difficult.

I took Karen and the boys to TGI Fridays one afternoon for lunch. After making our way into the restaurant we waited at the front near the reservation desk to be seated. There was no hostess to greet us--we stood and waited, and then waited some more.

I still feel self-conscious wheeling Karen into a public place. I'm not sure I will ever get to the point where I feel comfortable stationed behind that chair. The longer we waited, as waitresses rushed by and other customers were being served, the more embarrassed and irritated I became. After standing there for about seven or eight minutes I finally called out to one of the waitresses, "Hey is there any possibility of being seated in this place?" She knew from the tone of my voice that I was restless and irritated with the situation. A waiter finally came and escorted us to a table. By this time I was irritable and short-tempered, which is not a pleasant state to find oneself in. After all, going out for lunch is suppose to be a pleasant experience. Later in the course of the meal the manager came to our table to apologize. It seems they were a little short-handed that day.

Things like that happen. If I had been waiting to be seated or even if the boys had been with me I don't believe I would have lost my temper quite so easily. However, when I am out with my invalid wife I expect businesses and their staff to go out of their way to be extra courteous.

This unpleasant situation at TGI Fridays could have been avoided if I had planned ahead by making a simple telephone call. I would have been told the approximate seating time, I could have gotten handicapped accessibility information and would have in the long run avoided an unpleasant situation.

Another sure way to avoid a problem is to have the patient wait in the car while you go into the restaurant to check everything out. This will give you the opportunity to tell the hostess that you will need special seating for a handicapped person. This will generally resolve any kinks that might arise in the seating process.

Be wary of overcrowded restaurants. It's much more difficult to maneuver a wheelchair, which makes me nervous. The patient will become over anxious in this situation, as well. We have learned that by going early or later than the customary luncheon or dinner hour solves this problem nicely.

Another restaurant we enjoy frequenting is Cracker Barrel. On several occasions the waitress has led us all the way across the dining area and placed us at a table that was situated between two other tables. Sliding a person in a wheelchair between two tables can be extremely difficult. In situations like these you must learn to speak up and say, "I don't like this location. I don't like this tight spot. Will you please put us in another section." This simple request can make the difference between an unpleasant afternoon and a good day out.

The summer of 1995 found us in Myrtle Beach, South Carolina. My kids have always enjoyed going to the Hard Rock Cafe, and it just so happened that a new Hard Rock Cafe had just opened that week. As with the opening of any new trendy restaurant the lines were unbelievably long. I wheeled Karen to the end of the line and asked the man in front of me, if he knew how long it would be before we could be seated. His response was, "Well we were just told it could be up to two hours."

I couldn't believe my ears! There was no way I could stand out in the August heat with Karen for two hours. People with MS don't do well in the heat. Heat fatigues them quickly.

I had almost decided to load everybody back in the car, when I decided to check the timetable with one of the restaurant employees. I pushed Karen past the long line of people to the front entrance and asked how long our wait would be. The reply was, "None whatsoever, come on in." I couldn't believe my ears. We were taken in; shown an elevator and within fifteen minutes we were at a table with menus in our hands.

I can't tell you how incredibly good this made us feel. It was such a blessing to my family. This policy has been the norm at every Hard Rock Cafe we have been to. I am very pleased too say.

Another restaurant that has gone out of its way to give us immediate seating and courteous service is Planet Hollywood. The waiter made sure we were cared for and properly seated with as little hassle as possible.

I couldn't close a chapter about going out to eat without mentioning the fast food restaurant. Fast food chains can be difficult because so many of them have permanent tables and chairs. Almost all do have access ramps for the handicapped but conditions are cramped once you are inside. Karen's chair is usually placed at the end of the table, which means she inevitably blocks the aisle.

One way we have found to enjoy fast food restaurants is to use the drive-up window. On a mild day we find it a treat to order from the drive-up and then enjoy our meal in a park or some other scenic part of Newburgh.

I know it can be difficult and sometimes just a plain hassle taking an invalid out to a restaurant. Don't stay home and never go out. There's too much life to be lived for that. Lunch or dinner out on a routine basis will give the patient something to look forward too. They will have a much better attitude about their situation if they can get out and do something they enjoy.

The fact that restaurants and buildings today are handicapped accessible is a mark that our society has developed some sensitivity to the plight of the wheelchair bound individual. We still have a long way to go but at least these are issues that are no longer swept under the rug.

Chapter 30

Patience

The caregiver lives in an atmosphere conducive to impatience. People can lecture you as much and as often as they want about exercising patience, but they have no first hand knowledge of what it is to care for a chronically ill person day in and day out. Advice is always easier to give, than to take.

Care giving is a twenty-four hour a day examination of your ability to bend with pressure and to put your needs second to the patient.

You love the patient and gladly want to help them as much as possible. But there are days when you may have been awake a good part of the night because your loved one was ill, or needed you to help them turn over, or assist them to the restroom. You decide to try for a quick nap, and just as you are about to drop off, you are summoned by the patient to perform another task. This is a very unwelcome interruption; all you want is one hour for a nap. You grudgingly get up and comply with the request, but not necessarily with a smile on your lips or a pleasant disposition.

You may be watching your favorite television program when suddenly you are needed to help the care receiver to the bathroom or bring something to their chair. It feels as if you've already performed these same tasks at least fifty times during the day. Is it any wonder that you begin to feel irritable and out of sorts?

Impatience surfaces when I am pressed for time. There are mornings when I am in a hurry to leave the house and get to my office. I may be facing a deadline or just have a lot to do. Hurriedly I help Karen into her wheelchair; give her a quick bath; throw some clothes on her and I'm out the door.

There have been occasions when I left Karen sitting in the van while I ran a quick errand because it is such an ordeal to get her into the wheelchair, wheel her around the store and then load her back into the van.

Sometimes I feel like I am the only person in America who has to take their spouse to work with them. Sunday morning is a tough time in our house. I have the pressure of delivering a sermon to a congregation. There are people to see and things to do at my church. But before I leave the house I must make sure Karen is ready to go. When I feel impatient I rush about the house and nag Karen to hurry. And I know I am not smiling through the process.

The words, "I'm sorry," are not healing words for every problem but they will communicate to your loved one that you are aware that they have feelings. When I have snapped at Karen, I have to say, "I'm sorry I barked at you." The words, "I'm sorry," will not change the fact I was short-tempered, but it will help to defuse the situation. A willingness to admit failure goes a long way toward resolving hurt feelings and more unkind words.

It takes more than words. It takes a demonstration of patience. Set aside plenty of time for the care receiver. I could never get to church on Sunday morning if we waited until 8:00 a.m. to start getting dressed. I am up by 5:00 a.m. and Karen is up by 6:30 a.m. This allowance of time goes a long way in alleviating extra stress and frustration.

You will find that you have a kinder more patient disposition if you plan brief moments just for yourself and your own peace of mind. Go for a walk, arrange an hour at the gym, find someone to relieve you for a trip to the mall. But mostly importantly, patience comes through prayer. Pray a lot. Talk to God. Focus yourself and your thoughts on His inner strength. "The Fruit of the Spirit is Patience," (Galatians 5:22).

Chapter 31

Fear

What does "to fear," mean to you? The answer to that question is as individual as the person asked.

Some people fear failure. Some of us fear ridicule and censure. The aging beauty looks into the mirror and fears the reflection gazing back at her. The athlete fears the passing of time and the lost prowess of his youth. The elderly watch fearfully as their family and friends one by one depart this world, leaving them with only solitude and their memories. I ask you again, "What do you fear?"

In 1978 Karen and I left Dayton, Ohio for central Kentucky so I could pastor a church closer to Southern Baptist Theological Seminary where I was a student.

The move was difficult for Karen. This was the first time she had been away from her family and she had to give up a teaching position in Englewood, a suburban area outside of Dayton.

Naturally as soon as we were settled into our new home Karen started job hunting. The first job she found was at a daycare center operated by one of the local churches.

Karen came home crying after only a few hours at the daycare. There have only been a couple of times that Karen has buried her head in my arms and wept. This was one of those times. I can hear her sobs now. "Glenn I just couldn't stay there. It was the worst managed place. The ladies working there were doing nothing to watch the children. The kids were totally uncontrollable. It was the dirtiest place I have ever been. I just couldn't stay there," she sobbed.

I sensed the fear in her voice that day. She was afraid I would be disappointed in her.

The chronically ill fear disease, pain, disability, loneliness and death. As a caregiver and husband I hurt when Karen hurts. It breaks my heart when she cries. I feel her fear. And her fear is what multiple sclerosis is doing to her. I have held her in my arms and told her, "You don't deserve this disease. You have been too good a person. Nobody deserves this. I will help you every way I possibly can. I am here for you. I love you. I want to take care of you."

Karen has digressed to the point where she needs to have her legs exercised. Imagine yourself sitting for a week without moving your legs.

A hot bath relieves much of the pressure she experiences from being in one position for extended periods of time. Karen of course is unable to get in or out of the bathtub. So I must lift her from the wheelchair and place her in the water. I routinely go back and check on her every five to ten minutes.

One evening after I had helped Karen into the bath the boys and I started watching a movie. We became so engrossed in the plot that we lost all sense of time.

We were startled by a series of shrieking screams from the bathroom. "Uh oh, Mom's panicking," I told the boys. I rushed into the bathroom and found Karen frantically sobbing and panic-stricken. The water had been drained from the tub and she was sitting there with a towel wrapped around her almost hysterical.

I got her into her wheelchair and reassured her she was okay. Then she told me she was afraid we had left and had forgotten she was in the tub. Sobbing she said, "It is just so awful to be so afraid." I took her into my arms and she wept like a child. My heart was broken and I cried with her. "Glenn," she said, "you just don't realize what it is like to be so dependent. I can't get myself out of the tub. I can't do anything for myself. You don't realize what a scary feeling that is, to be so dependent. I'm so afraid of what is going to happen to me. I don't want to get worse. I don't want to be an invalid. I am so afraid of where this is taking me. I'm not afraid of death. Death would be simple. I'm afraid of being totally bedridden. I am afraid of being unable to feed myself. I'm so tired of being afraid."

In Karen's case she knows where she will spend eternity. Her confidence in God and her home in heaven has never been questioned. Karen has been dedicated to God her entire life. She doesn't fear death or eternity. She fears the process. The unknown and just how far the disease will progress are frightening to her. It is frightening for all of us who love her.

The caregiver struggles to help the patient through the fears of their illness. It is not easy. You pray with them. You cry with them. You worship with them. You help them. You do your best to convey to them that you are there to help and that you aren't going to leave them.

Chapter 32

Trying Everything

It is the nature of our species, to fight for survival, to cling tenaciously to life. And so it is with Karen. She is a young woman with two young children she loves very much. She has a lot to live for. In her battle with multiple sclerosis we have tried almost every drug, vitamin, injection, potion, tonic, and treatment available.

I have already discussed Beta Interferon, Avonex and Copaxon in previous chapters. At this point in MS treatment they are the big three drugs that MS patients are trying in hopes of being helped. All three drugs are currently incredibly expensive. In the case of all three of these medications Karen tried them all and continued to decline.

A couple of years ago we received a cassette tape from an acquaintance. This tape contained the testimonials of several people who had allegedly been cured of multiple sclerosis. This cure was affected by the ingestion of vitamins. The testimonials were glowing and very inspiring, so we attended several meetings that the company representatives hosted. These meetings were almost like rallies. The purpose of these seminars was to enlist people to sell the vitamins.

More money could be made by the salesperson if they enlisted other people, and so on, forming a pyramid effect.

We tried the vitamins for several months. They were good vitamins. But we soon discovered we could go to the grocery store and buy the same vitamins for a fraction of the cost.

Cantron is another multivitamin that was recommended to us as a cure for multiple sclerosis. The distributor of this product contacted us, and for several weeks, repeatedly called our home telephone number to extol the benefits of this amazing product. Testimonials from people who had apparently been cured or helped by Cantron were sent to us. Karen took this product for several months. Like any other vitamin or mineral supplement it was good for her, but it did nothing to alleviate the progression of the disease.

We have in the past and will continue to take vitamin supplements. Vitamins are a valuable adjunct for those of us who are forced to eat on the run or perhaps don't eat the balanced diet that we should. But in our experience, vitamin supplements did not slow the progression of multiple sclerosis.

Karen and I received a very excited telephone call from her parents in Dayton, Ohio. They had just heard some wonderful reports on the effectiveness of magnets. These magnets had supposedly originated in Japan. The idea behind the magnet theory was that the MS would be drawn out of her body. And as with all the other alternative treatments we had tried, there were many glowing testimonials from people who had been helped or cured of multiple sclerosis. The distributor in Dayton sent us a mattress for Karen to sleep on and a cushion for her back to try on a trial basis. After several months it became apparent to us that the magnets were having no effect. Luckily we did not purchase the mattress and chair pads. It would have been an expenditure of more than five hundred dollars.

The sad reality is there is no cure for multiple sclerosis. Another reality is that MS effects everybody differently. What works for one person may be absolutely useless to someone else.

In many cases, people with MS will have a spontaneous remission. Jimmy Grayson, a good friend of mine, told of his wife having a tremendous remission. "One day she got up and just started walking. We thought God had healed her. In time she went back to teaching school and we had our second child. But then one day it came back."

I believe wholeheartedly that the remissions many people experience coincide with some therapy they are trying. But who can say what triggers a remission? As of this writing there is very little help available to sufferers of MS who are chronic progressive.

In Karen's quest for healing she has tried physical therapy, swimming, and counseling.

Karen has sought the help and advice of several counselors. I believe the counseling has been a positive experience for her. We never believed the counseling could alter the course of the disease, but for her mental health it has been most worthwhile.

At the end of this long list of medications and treatments, the most valuable and the most helpful therapy we have found to date is prayer. Karen has prayed. We have prayed together. Our families have prayed. The church I pastor is a praying church.

We have allowed and welcomed the laying on of hands. She has been surrounded by small, loving circles of friends who have prayed fervently to the Lord for her healing. Karen has been anointed with oil and prayed for. She is on the prayer lists of several churches. I have four male friends who meet with me every Thursday morning at six o'clock for prayer. We spend twenty to thirty minutes in prayer and always pray for my wife.

I have been to gatherings that Karen could not attend and have had people pray for Karen by placing their hands on me as a point of contact. They prayed for her healing as they touched me. It was a moving experience.

I understand God does not always answer prayer the way we would have Him to. He does not always say yes. Sometimes God says no. Sometimes God says wait awhile. And then there are days when God is silent.

The Bible talks about prayer. Jesus prayed. He prayed for his followers. He prayed for Himself (John 17). Before He was crucified He prayed in agony in the garden of Gethsemane. "Going a little farther, he fell to the ground and prayed that if possible the hour might pass from Him, 'Abba, Father,' he said, 'everything is possible for you. Take this cup from me. Yet not what I will, but what You will,'" (Mark 14:35-36). He prayed if possible that the cross he was about to bear and the death he would die might be removed from Him. In other words, "God, if it's possible let me escape this death on the cross." But God did not remove that terrible ordeal of crucifixion from Jesus.

God does not remove the terrible ordeals from our lives either.

When we pray we need to pray as Jesus taught us to pray, "Thy will be done on earth as it is in heaven." This means we must be willing to accept what God's will is, and pray to that end for His will to be done.

For us the journey of this disease has been filled with lots of signs that have said, "Help is to the right. Hope is to the left. Healing is around the corner. Feeling better is just over the next mountain." When we finally arrived on the other side of that mountain we discovered that we were lost. The road we had traveled led only to frustration and dismay.

Chapter 33

There is Always Somebody Worse

I mourned the fact I had no shoes. And then I met a man who had no feet. How true that old cliché is, and how relevant to my life as a caregiver.

We can learn so much by observing those who are weathering life's hardships. It is important to take note of how they are managing, how they daily find the courage to face the world. So often we focus on ourselves. We see only ourselves. I think it is helpful to look around and realize that there are always people who have a greater burden to bear or a harder road to travel. I remind myself during times of darkness and despair, when Karen has had an especially difficult day that it could indeed be worse. "But there for the grace of God, go I."

I was pushing Karen through the mall not too long ago and saw a mother pushing her child in a wheelchair. The child was apparently born with a disability. The child appeared to be a teenage girl approximately seventeen years old, and very deformed. The mother appeared to be in her forties and very tired and care worn.

The wife of a dear friend was severely injured in a car crash, leaving her paralyzed. She is unable to do the simplest things for herself. We thank God every day that Karen still has the use of her hands and arms and can wheel her self about.

An attitude of thanksgiving and gratitude for the blessings we have been given can mean the difference between a life filled with frustration and self-pity, and a life that is truly lived to the fullest. There are people living in very small houses on meager fixed incomes that have a thankful spirit and manage very happily with what they have. There are people living in wealthy neighborhoods, driving expensive cars who spend their time in bitterness lamenting what they do not have.

A thankful attitude, a grateful heart, it's all up to you. It's within your power to look around you and see just how very fortunate and blessed you are.

Am I making light of your affliction? Am I chastising you or trying to shame you? No dear friend. I would never presume to such a thing. Your pain is genuine, just as Karen's pain and my pain are genuine. Watching the unfortunate mother wheel her deformed child through the mall does not diminish Karen's ordeal or the pain I experience as her husband.

Let us look to those who have suffered greatly and yet have never lost hope in the ultimate goodness of the Lord that we may be challenged and inspired to carry our own burdens with hope and dignity.

Chapter 34

Who Would Have Thought

The first time I saw Jimmy Grayson was when I attended The First Baptist Church in Inez, Kentucky. Jimmy was a big guy about 6'1 and weighed at least 250 pounds. He welcomed me warmly and congratulated me on my decision to become a Christian.

Jimmy baptized me that night. From that time forward he became not only a steadfast pastor and friend, but also an example of what a good and faithful caregiver should be.

I never dreamed as a fifteen-year-old boy that I was seeing my own reflection mirrored in Jimmy Grayson and his wife Evelyn. Jimmy was a pastor. I would become a pastor. His wife had multiple sclerosis and was in a wheelchair. I would marry a girl who would be stricken with multiple sclerosis and become wheelchair bound.

A lady once said to me, "Glenn you must have prayed once to become just like Jimmy Grayson. And it looks like the Lord answered your prayers."

I don't know how Jimmy made it really. He was committed to caring for Evelyn. I never heard him complain. He took care of Evelyn for more years than I know. I met them in 1970. She was in a wheelchair then. It must have been an incredibly long and difficult road for the both of them.

For sixteen years Jimmy lived about five feet behind the church he served. He had almost no privacy. He parked his car beneath the carport attached to his house. People always knew when Jimmy was at home. He was totally accessible to everyone. I think after years of caring for Evelyn and the members of his congregation the strain became too much. Jimmy began to experience severe heart problems and had grave difficulties with diabetes, almost losing a leg to the disease.

Looking back I know I felt too comfortable knocking on Jimmy's door. I just loved him and so did everyone else. He always believed in me and encouraged me. Once in Paintsville, Kentucky I pointed to a large Baptist church and asked, "Brother Jimmy, do you think I will ever pastor a church as big as that one?"

Looking at me and expressing himself as only this big guy could; he lifted his hand and pointed his finger at me and said, "Far bigger than that son! Far bigger than that!"

His amazingly positive attitude as a caregiver is something I will never forget. He never complained about his wife's illness and all the stress I know he experienced as a caregiver.

We never know when we should be taking mental notes as we journey through life. Sometimes we are witnessing actual situations we may be confronted with. I think people like Jimmy and Evelyn Grayson are gifts from God.

Chapter 35

How is Karen Doing?

Many people have prayed for Karen's health. They would love to think their prayers have been answered and so would I. They wait in anticipation for a good report. I wish I could give it to them. I have never faulted anyone for showing concern, but the question, "How is Karen doing?" asked over and over again is emotionally draining. Every time I have to rehash Karen's illness it depletes a little more of my energy.

There is nothing new to report. There was a period of time when we were trying drugs, water therapy and a number of alternative treatments. When asked about Karen's condition, I could report, "Now we're trying Beta Interferon." I could say, "We are now trying a new vitamin." But that is no longer the case, we have depleted all our options. The stark truth is that my wife is slowly but steadily declining, not very pleasant for the casual acquaintance to hear.

Imagine if you will, walking into your place of employment, and before you had even removed your coat and hat, fifty people walk up to you and inquire about the health of a sick loved one. This does not happen occasionally but on a regular basis. The longer you deal with this situation the harder it becomes.

As time passes a certain amount of resentment and antagonism towards the so-called well meaning questioner develops. This resentment soon turns to anger. I must bite my tongue to keep from blurting out, "That's stupid! Why would anyone ask such an ignorant question? Buddy, do you know and understand that my wife has MS? Do you see she is in the wheelchair? Sir, why would you ask, 'How is Karen doing?' Isn't it obvious?"

Do I sound harsh to you? Or do you, as a caregiver, understand exactly how frustrated I have been by the eternal question, "How is Karen doing?" Perhaps you too know how difficult it is to answer this question.

I must reply in some fashion or be considered rude. Most of the time I simply say, "Just fine." This will usually suffice. The well-meaning acquaintance can then feel satisfied and move on. The difficulty arises when they won't take "just fine" for an answer. They follow one question with another. "She is getting better then?" To which I must truthfully reply, "No, she is in reality a little worse." Now everyone is uncomfortable.

There are several reasons people feel compelled to ask this question. The casual acquaintance may ask, "How is

Karen doing," out of politeness. They know Karen as a church member or simply as my wife. They feel it is the Christian thing to do, so they inquire about her health. Quite often they do not really want an honest answer to their question. Can you imagine the shocked expression on someone's face if I honestly replied, "Karen is having a really difficult time. She's getting worse every day. The numbness is moving into her hands and arms and her sight is deteriorating more all the time. She has almost no control over her bladder. We have to change her clothes constantly. And worst of all she is in horrible pain from a huge, open pressure sore on her hip." Do you think the average person just trying to make polite conversation would appreciate an answer like that? Neither do I.

Many people are under the impression that I expect them to ask how my wife is. So, out of a sense of duty, they will pose the question. I do not fault them for this assumption, but I do not expect anyone to ask about Karen's well being out of a sense of duty.

There are people who ask me how Karen is because they have nothing better to say. They don't really know me but feel they must make conversation. This puts an unwelcome burden upon me. I would much prefer discussing the weather, sports, politics, anything except, "How is Karen doing?"

Of course many people ask about Karen's health out of genuine love and concern. They are longing to hear that she is improving. I wish with all my heart that she were. No matter who poses the question, the result is the same; I am mentally and emotionally exhausted.

As a caregiver I deal with my wife's illness seven days a week, fifty-two weeks a year. I can't express to you how difficult it was when Karen was taking Beta Interferon and was depressed and angry with me and the world in general. It was an incredible strain to smile and tell everyone Karen was "just fine" after spending weeks on end dressing her, bathing her and caring for her only to be berated and verbally abused. How I longed to hear the question, "How's Glenn doing?"

I must confess, perhaps it was for the best that during those terrible times dealing with Karen's mood swings, I wasn't asked, "How's Glenn doing?" I might have said, "Buddy, I am tired. I am sick and tired. I am emotionally beat down. Do you know how hard it is to dress somebody and bathe her when you have been given a verbal wherewithal? And buddy, this has been going on a long time. And it looks like the worst is yet to come. Now does that give you any clue how I'm doing?"

I need a break just like anyone else. When I walk into the church door I need the spiritual nourishment of worship just as much as any member of my congregation. Spending what small time I have for worship rehashing what I have had to deal with all week is not a spiritual break.

I decided after much deliberation to write an article for the church newsletter addressing this situation. The results were very positive. I feared some of my membership might not understand my feelings. The next Sunday after the article appeared dozens from my congregation told me they appreciated knowing how I felt. Several even apologized for the many times they had persistently asked about Karen.

As a caregiver you must deal with this question in your own way and fashion. I have personally found writing out a statement of no more than two or three lines on an index card to be most helpful. When someone pops the question about the patient, you simply hand him or her the card. This may sound strange. But it is really quite effective and as the condition of the patient changes you can update the information on the card.

It is also helpful to tell some of your trusted friends about how upsetting you find constant questions about the patient's health to be. They can then pass your views along to others.

I have always found it helpful to take the lead in the conversation. You may wish to discuss sports, or national news. Guide the conversation away from discussing the care receiver.

You can try hiding. Hiding is effective for a while. But I don't recommend it. In the long run the caregiver is the one who is hurt. We need to be able to come and go freely. Hiding out and ducking around corners is an added burden none of us needs.

There is no easy way to deal with this situation. But deal with it you must, for your own stability and peace of mind.

Chapter 36

Try to Understand

Karen spent years preparing to be a schoolteacher. She loved her profession as much as life itself. She completed a degree in music with an emphasis in piano. She later earned a master's degree in education adding the needed endorsements to teach kindergarten through twelfth grade. The last seven years before she was forced to give up her career was spent as a counselor at the elementary level. At the age of thirty-five Karen looked forward to a long productive career in education.

Karen loved the elementary school environment. She worked long hours preparing lesson plans and going over class assignments. It was very important to Karen to be thoroughly prepared when she walked through the classroom door to greet her students. Karen gave it her all because she loved teaching so much. It was her life.

And then multiple sclerosis struck. Slowly, but inevitably the disease took its toll. Karen found herself tired and exhausted, barely able to make it through the school day. She began to limp. The stairs at her school became a major obstacle. It was becoming more and more difficult for her to hobble up and down those stairs to change classrooms. Teaching had become a major chore instead of the delight it had once been.

It wasn't an easy decision for Karen to give up teaching. After several months of soul searching Karen came to the realization that she no longer had the stamina necessary to continue as an elementary school teacher. Karen requested a temporary leave of absence. Applying for temporary disability made the decision to leave teaching much easier for Karen.

We had high hopes that her condition would improve with the aid of therapy and medication. It was always understood that when her health improved Karen would resume her teaching career exactly where she'd left off.

Our hopes for a remission have been dashed one by one. At this point nothing shy of a miracle wrought from God would enable Karen to once again re-enter the classroom. And yes we do believe in miracles.

Watching Karen struggle with MS and knowing she will never be able to do that which she loves, teach has been heartbreaking for me. When we care for the elderly we know they have had the opportunity to live their lives. They have worked, raised a family and retired. They were afforded their chance, as it were. When someone is deprived of health in the midstream of life it rips away those opportunities.

I know Karen has been an inspiration to many of my parishioners. I feel very strongly that my church has become a more caring and prayerful community of believers as they witnessed Karen's struggle. I know they pray for me as a struggling pastor and beleaguered husband and father. I know they pray for Karen and God's healing Grace and I know they pray for our children.

I feel blessed by their prayers as I struggle to be a good caregiver. I never dreamed that I would be faced with such a daunting challenge. Multiple sclerosis has severely tested my Christianity. It has only been by the Grace of God that I have been able to withstand the trials of Karen's illness and the pressures of a caregiver.

As I look back upon the life I had with my family before Karen's illness I see that what I considered to be struggles and hardships were really nothing in comparison to what we are battling now. I watched Karen give up a career she loved, just as other caregivers have had to stand by and watch their loved ones struggling and sacrificing.

I know in my heart that nothing is permanent. Life is temporary. All that we own is temporary. I have a closet full of clothes that someday will go to someone who can use them. My house will be lived in someday by either my children or someone else. My automobiles are eventually headed for the junk pile. Our possessions are not forever. Our lives are not forever. Our relationships are not forever. Marriage may last a lifetime but then it ends. Whatever bad or good things come our way are temporary.

Realizing that life and all that we own is not forever does not make it easier for the loved one who sees life changing before their eyes. We don't count on such unwelcome change as ill health coming to us in our youth. Poor health is for the person in his or her late seventies or eighties. I never dreamed of having a wife in a wheelchair at the age of forty-two. This is a demonstration to me anew and afresh that there are no guarantees to longevity or good health. Again, it is vital that we cherish each day and all that we have.

Chapter 37

The Dying Process

Multiple sclerosis gives a person ample time to prepare for death; this disease does not afford a quick and easy demise. No, the loved one wastes away little by little, month by month, day by day. The chronic progressive patient may linger as long as fifteen or twenty years before death finally comes. It is a long, very long goodbye.

I find myself in the unbearable situation of watching my wife daily losing ground, fading away to a mere shadow of her former self. So often people will ask, "Is Karen any worse? Has there been any change?" I do not notice change on a daily basis, or even a monthly basis. But in hindsight, I can look back over the last six months to a time when Karen was still able to get in and out of the bathtub unaided. Or I can think back to four months ago when Karen was still able to stand so as to slip a pair of slacks over her hips. This is how I measure the progression of the disease. When I think back over the months and years since the diagnosis, I can see quite clearly the toll that Karen has had to pay. Her pain is felt keenly and acutely by all those who her love her.

Watching someone you love who complains of feeling a little "strange" digress to having vision problems, numbness in the legs and feet, slurred speech, lost function of their hands and arms to eventually being unable to breathe, is cruel and hard. Multiple sclerosis comes in waves; it is like watching a boxer, pinned against the ropes, receive a devastating blow with no time to recover his wits. He is hit again hard; this blow depletes his strength further. The hits keep coming--they never stop. There is nothing the boxer can do to save himself, just as there is nothing the sufferer of multiple sclerosis can do to save themselves. All that is left is to watch your loved one slowly lose a little more function, a little more mobility, they become weaker, dying inch by inch.

The knowledge that someone you love and care for has a disease that will eventually bring about his or her death isn't easy for anyone to accept. Once the initial shock of this revelation has lessened, you are in a position to make adjustments and act accordingly.

This means talking to your children. I think one of the hardest things I have ever had to do in my life was talk to the kids about the possibility of their mother dying.

In May of 1997, Karen had what the doctor described as a seizure. Karen was rushed to the hospital. The boys and I waited outside the emergency room entrance. We had no idea at the time what was going on. We were terrified we might be losing Karen. We talked about what would happen if mommy didn't make it. Naturally the boys were frightened. They weren't prepared to give up a mother any more than I was prepared to give up my wife.

The tragedy with the children is that Zachary does not remember a time when his mother wasn't fighting for her life. Zachary has vague memories of his mother taking him to first grade, but even then Karen was limping badly, dragging her right leg. It was during this time that Karen made the decision to ask for a temporary leave of absence from her teaching position. The fatigue and the daily climb up and down the stairs had become too much.

Jared was in the fourth grade when his mother made the decision to stop teaching. His memory of her as a vital, active woman is certainly clearer than Zachary's is. It has been very difficult for the boys to see their mother go from a healthy schoolteacher to a woman who is obliged to spend a great deal of time in a wheelchair or on the couch in desperate need of rest. As the years slip by we have watched wife and mother slowly, very slowly become just a shadow of what she once was.

The slow death process means talking to the extended family as well. In our society we generally try to ignore the subject of dying. But the parents of the patient and other loved ones need to be a part of this conversation. This is their child. They need to fully understand the course of the disease and what the ultimate outcome will be. This does not mean that the patient has given up on medicine or prayer. On the contrary, every attempt to get well should be made. It means that you the caregiver, the patient and the family members understand what you are dealing with.

The caregiver at some point needs to take advantage of the opportunity in a gracious gentle way to talk to the patient about their funeral wishes. The care receiver will appreciate this opportunity for expression. They may not want to talk about their funeral because at the time it may seem very unimportant. When you are selecting caskets or making funeral arrangements or deciding on a burial place you will be so grateful that you had this little talk. Furthermore, write down some notes. Find a safe place to store these notes-- you'll be so glad you did.

A discussion about the children's future needs to take place. What would the patient's wishes be? What would they like to see happen five years into the future about the kid's college education? This does not guarantee the fulfillment of those wishes. Times and circumstances change, there needs to be an attitude that when the time comes everybody will have to do what is best in the given situation. However, it will be very beneficial to be able to look back and say, "This is what Karen wanted." Or, "This is what Karen would have done."

Talk to your spouse or loved one about a living will. A living will is vital to anyone with a disease like multiple sclerosis. The living will states the wishes of the patient in the event that they are no longer able to speak for themselves. This will also be a blessing to the caregiver. You will have a great many emotional issues to deal with. It is incredibly draining to watch someone die before your eyes. The living will expresses the patient's desire that they do not wish to be kept on any kind of life support system indefinitely.

There are many cases where patients suffering from Alzheimer's have been kept on a feeding tube or similar life-preserving device for months or even longer. A living will allows the patient to choose how their last days will be spent. They can determine if they want to be kept alive via machines and artificial means or if they want to go on to their eternity in peace.

As the patient declines you will find yourself faced with many new tasks. For example, just placing Karen in her wheelchair has changed over the last several months. The development of a pressure sore on her hip now needs extra care and attention. After I dress Karen, if she has the strength to elevate herself by placing her hands on the arms of her chair and pushing up, I slide a pillow behind her back and onto the seat of the wheelchair.

Placing the pillow on the seat of her chair is a small, almost trivial task. The trivial tasks add up. Being a caregiver is not about one simple task. It is about hundreds of little tasks, snowballing, until you feel completely overwhelmed.

I suppose a disease of the magnitude of multiple sclerosis makes one long for the good old days, to remember the past when Karen was on the move and was very alive and active. We thought it was so awful when she first experienced vision problems. We were traumatized when she had to use a walker for balance. Little did we know how wonderful those days were in comparison to where we are now. I have often looked back and thought how great it would be if we could just go back four years. Or, if we could go back six months, she was certainly much stronger then.

I have asked myself the question, "What will tomorrow bring? Will tomorrow mean that she will no longer be able to sit in her wheelchair? Will tomorrow mean she will have to be fed because her hands and arms will not function?"

The answers to these questions will only be told by time and the heartbreaking realization that, yes these continuing declines will most likely occur. They will force us to look back with longing for this moment, just as we long for other past moments.

I have learned to give thanks for the blessings of today, because tomorrow will likely be worse, or for Karen, there may not be a tomorrow. Please forgive me if this sounds horribly negative and pessimistic, but baring a miracle from God, this is our reality.

Chapter 38

FOR KAREN

The Grand Piano

There is a beautiful grand piano that rests quietly in our family room. The musician who played it is still living in the house. But everything is different now. Karen has given it up. She avoids the piano and understandably so.

The piano contributed so much to her life and identity. She perfected this instrument. It obeyed her every command. There was nothing her mind could conceive of, no musical score so complex, that her talented hands could not transform into a work of beauty and splendor.

Karen's piano has traveled with us from church to church and house to house. When we were living in Northern Kentucky I was called to pastor The First Baptist Church of Pikeville, Kentucky. Karen wasn't happy about leaving her teaching position and pulling up stakes to move to Pikeville, but she loved me and as a caring wife wanted to support my career move.

To ease the transition and to say thank you I purchased a beautiful ebony Kiwai piano for Karen. The piano adorned our house in Pikeville and later our home in Louisa, Kentucky.

The piano now sits, untouched in a place of honor in our family room, an ever-present reminder to me, and of course to Karen, of days gone by. I remember gatherings of family and friends circled around the piano. Karen would play the accompaniment and we would all sing off key. Those were some very happy days.

Karen can't play the piano anymore. Multiple sclerosis has robbed her hands of the agility and strength she needs to strike the keys. I feel great remorse when I think of her working and practicing every day of her childhood to perfect her musical skills.

By her senior year of college Karen had mastered the piano. Her senior recital was a grand performance to match no other. Karen had the ability and talent to have been a concert pianist.

During the first year of our marriage, Karen became the pianist for The Far Hills Baptist Church in Dayton, Ohio. Far Hills is the largest Baptist Church in Ohio with an attendance of over one thousand people every Sunday morning. Karen was paid thirty-eight dollars a week for playing at Far Hills. She would drive over on Sunday morning and return for the evening service Sunday night.

Likewise she made the trip on Wednesday for choir rehearsal and services. That says a lot about her love and dedication to the church and to her art.

One day shortly after we had moved to Newburgh, I was working in the garage when something caught my attention and made me stop what I was doing. I heard the faint sound of music coming from inside the house. Slowly one note would ring out and then another. It sounded like a first year piano student laboriously searching for the correct keys to play. I hung my head and wept. My heart was breaking. The vision of my wife tentatively and painstakingly striking the keys of her piano, an instrument that she had mastered and played with such artistry and grace was too much to bear.

Karen knows, through no fault of her own, that she will never be able to play the piano again. Knowing this doesn't make it any easier. It's a reality that has been very hard for her and for me to accept. We don't like changes. We especially do not like the changes that are forced upon us or that are beyond our control.

I learned life can change very quickly. The freedom we have to run, walk, play an instrument, and work at our chosen profession can be stripped away from us in a matter of seconds.

When I was sixteen my father helped me buy my first car, a brown Chevy Chevelle. My father allowed me the freedom and privilege to drive my car to school. In November of 1971 I found myself in the hospital with a dislocated hip and facial lacerations. Driving too fast down a country road and almost killing myself had changed my life.

For a while I was forced to give up many of the things I enjoyed. I missed most of my junior year of high school basketball. I no longer had a car, so I rode the school bus.

In time my hip healed and I was able to put down the crutches and walk normally. Those things I enjoyed doing slowly became possible for me again. For the person suffering from MS or some other chronic debilitating disease the freedom to do what they love most will never return.

Understanding, remembering and appreciating all that your loved one had and has lost is crucial. Karen has given up everything. Amidst all the emotional turmoil she has experienced because of medications and drugs, she has been able on most days to go to her Bible and pray for the strength to make it through the day with her disease. Karen at times exhibits a peace that can only come from God. Jesus said, "Peace I leave with you; my peace I give you. I do not give to you as the world gives. Do not let your hearts be troubled and do not be afraid" (John 15:27).

In Sickness and in Health

Karen and I stood in front of the altar on December 20, 1975 at the old Crestview Baptist Church. The Reverend Delano McMinn and a pastoral friend, David White presided over the wedding ceremony.

"I Glenn, take thee Karen to be my wedded wife. To have and to hold from this day forward; for better for worse; for richer for poorer; in sickness and in health; to love and to cherish till death do us part; and forsaking all others I will be faithful unto you so long as we both shall live."

As a twenty-year-old college student, I don't think I could fully comprehend or measure the breath or the depth of the marriage vows. They were just beautiful poetic words I repeated as so many other grooms before me had.

I have been an ordained minister for twenty-five years and have performed many weddings. I have talked at length with couples entering into the marriage contract. I often find in our pre-wedding planning session that very little has been discussed about the wedding ceremony, per se.

There has been a lot of discussion about sex, finances, housing, children and child rearing. But very little time or thought has gone into the wedding vows. Here we have two people prepared to stand before God and give their sacred pledge to one another, yet they rarely take the time or trouble to fully examine what lies behind the words, "For better or worse."

"For better or worse," it begs the question, "How bad or how worse?" The spouse who is caring for a chronically ill husband or wife learns first hand what "For better or for worse" really means.

When I uttered those words I was making a firm commitment. I promised Karen to do my best. In times of want and hardship I would be at her side, just as I had been at her side during times of plenty.

Pretty words, easily said, not so easily lived. Marriage is wonderful when everything is going well; the family has a good income, the children are well behaved, but what happens to this equation if the husband or wife becomes ill? The family income diminishes, the once well-behaved children now seem demanding and difficult and the marriage is no longer wonderful. It is work. It is very tedious hard work.

When we stand in front of the minister repeating the vows we are in a state of euphoria. We can't see past the happiness of the moment. So we glibly vow, "For better or for worse," never dreaming we might someday be put to the test.

If God had shown me a video of Karen's illness and all that we would have to endure, I would still have married her. I love her. I wouldn't have changed one syllable of our wedding vows, but I would have weighed each word more carefully and taken to heart the seriousness of what I was promising.

"For richer for poorer." The average American couple battles more about money, bills and finances than any other issue. We dream of richer. We fantasize about winning the lottery and striking it rich. Poverty is something no one aspires to. How many people do you know dream of losing all their wealth and becoming homeless? It's a foolish question. However, if you are a caregiver you may find yourself very close to this predicament.

Unfortunately, in this day and age, it seems that more and more families must have two incomes to survive. Before Karen's illness she taught school. We quickly became accustomed to a two-income lifestyle. Her job made it possible for us to own two vehicles, which meant two car payments. Her paycheck meant she could buy new clothes for both she and our two boys. Plus we were able to add to our savings for that rainy day.

What happens if the main breadwinner in the family is the one who becomes ill? In the beginning we are all convinced that, "Love will find a way to overcome all obstacles." But then the rent is due, and the phone bill, and the electric bill, and the car payment and there's nothing in the house to eat.

The caregiver has to either accept a lesser standard of living or be very wise with his or her money. This may mean moving from a large house to something smaller and more economical. It may very well mean that the spouse who never worked outside the home will have to seek employment. Or under some circumstances the caregiver and the patient may have to consider moving back home with parents.

"In sickness and in health." I've wept bitter tears over that simple phrase; had I only known what it really meant.

This vow is one that we cannot expect to fully understand until we have been called upon to put it into practice. When a loved one becomes desperately ill unto death, then the love for the person, the love of God and a desire to do the right thing must become paramount in our lives. I have a great need and find enormous comfort in Psalm 23:4 where David said; "Even though I walk through the valley of the shadow of death, I will fear no evil, for you are with me." I know the terrain of that valley very well. When someone you love is dying one day at a time it becomes a long valley with long, fearsome shadows. And the need of

God's sustaining Grace to protect us both from being overwhelmed with fear and despair, grows greater with each step of the journey.

"To love and to cherish," that's easy, especially if it's the honeymoon. The newlywed couple gaze into each other's eyes and say, "I will always love you." The wedding night is perfect. Karen was a feast for the eyes. The thought of loving her and holding her dear to my heart for the rest of my life filled me with joy.

Twenty years have past. And the woman I felt such love and passion for has become a mere shadow of who she once was. Instead of the scent of perfume there is the musty odor of illness and decay about her person. Her skin that was once soft and radiant is now covered with sores and wounds from falling or being scraped by a wheelchair. The woman with dreams and aspirations can only imagine what might have been.

I Glenn take thee Karen to be my wedded wife; to have and to hold from this day forward; for better for worse; for richer for poorer; in sickness and in health; to love and to cherish till death do us part.

"Till death do us part." I can state with absolute certainty that I had no idea the ramifications of "till death do us part," on my wedding day. I know now what it means.

Living out our vows is different than saying our vows. To say we are married until we die is saying regardless of what happens we will stay with the marriage relationship. Regardless of differences, hardship, incompatibility or sickness we will try to work it out and stay with each other until death separates us.

The last thing Karen did before we left to go on our honeymoon was to hug her dad. The last words I spoke to him were, "I will take care of her." Words. The words we say at the altar of marriage. The words we thoughtlessly toss about. "I will take care of her?" In my twenty-year old way, I meant that. I mean that today. If I had known what was ahead of us I would have said those words with great fear and trembling. When I say those words today, I say them knowing that only by God's Grace will I be able to take care of her.

Today I do not stay with Karen because of some words I said over twenty-three years ago in a ceremony. I stay with Karen because I love her and I stay with her because she is my wife. It's not easy surviving a long-term chronically progressive illness. It is a test of everyone's courage, faith and love. God enables us along this difficult unplanned for journey of life because He is our helper (Hebrews 13:6).

What's Next?

There is nothing for sure when it comes to multiple sclerosis. Life with this disease is an uncertain journey. Even though millions of people have suffered and eventually died from MS there is still much about this disease that researchers are trying to discover.

There is a chance that Karen may live many years. The possibility exists that the disease may progress faster and bring about her death. Who knows?

Should Karen become so ill that I am needed by her side I would take the time away from my career to be with her. Should she get to the point of death I would never in my wildest dreams be anywhere else but at her side.

We wait. We pray. We wonder what will happen next. We think, "It would be impossible for things to get worse and then they do."

There is no permanence in this world. Today is here and then it is gone. All that we have or know is never really constant. Keep your focus upon God. His love is never changing. His promises are faithful.

One Night

It is the evening; approximately 9:15 and the boys are brushing their teeth and preparing for bed. I am finishing up whatever project I have been working on and Karen is rolling into the eating area of our kitchen. It is about this way every night because Karen sees to it that the boys are in their places for their bedtime devotion and prayer.

Karen as always has a favorite book that she feels will be interesting to the boys. With trembling hands affected by the MS she slowing and carefully seeks to turn the page as she reads. Her voice is shaky at times and her word pronunciation sometimes unclear.

It is obvious that Karen likes to read. A habit she developed and grew to love as a child comes easily for her as two boys 12 and 15 settle in to listen to what she has to read.

It looks different to me in some way.

I think it is wonderful because I remember as a young child having someone read to me. But my boys are not tiny children; they are young men sitting at the table with an occasional yawn.

There is an occasional protest or two throughout the week about this nightly commitment to reading and prayer. But with heads sometimes upright and other times down on the table their eyes are focused and I know they are taking in every word.

Reading down the page it seems as though Karen's voice grows a little more stable. There is more strength to it as she pronounces her words with more clarity.

For the next fifteen minutes the boys listen and soon it is time to pray. Sometimes I'm asked to lead in prayer. "Daddy, you pray. You don't pray as long as mom," Zachary notes. I confess my prayers are probably quicker and to the point. I'm tired and ready for bed after a long day. My prayers kind of seem standard in this setting. "Dear God, thank you for this good day. Thank you for friends, our church and all that we have. Give us a good night's sleep. Watch over Jared and Zachary as they sleep. Lord help mommy to get better. In Jesus' name we pray, Amen."

But if Karen is praying, the prayer is a little slower and a little more intentional and often more specific concerning the cares and the needs of the day or the needs of the boys.

The prayer is over and there is a goodnight from all and a hug for mom. The boys go to bed and I head to our bedroom. For the next few minutes Karen can be heard wheeling her chair up to the kitchen sink and somehow managing to turn on the water and wash every dirty dish. The dryer door opens and Karen begins folding clothes for the

239

next day. And should I get up for a glass of orange juice before I drop off to sleep, she will be at the kitchen table with her Bible open doing a home Bible study assignment.

Going to bed with no idea how long she will try to stay up, I know Karen will soon wheel herself to our couch. She will make sure there is a cover and a liner over the sofa. She will then put on the brakes to her wheelchair and somehow manage to push herself off her chair and onto the sofa. For so long she has only been able to sleep on this sofa.

I find myself alone in bed. I'm alone. I'm lonely. I remember the nights and years of sleeping in the same bed with my wife. I'm tired because I have made myself that way. I have gone the entire day without stopping. I work, exercise, and run errands for Karen or my boys to fill up the day. Somehow it eases the pain.

Sleep is never all night. Four hours maybe five, six hours is a good night's sleep. But for the first few hours the sleep is deep from sheer exhaustion.

Suddenly I am awakened by a voice. It is the voice of someone crying. There is no mistaking this sound. It is Karen. I have heard her cry so many times, when she didn't know I was around the corner. I've heard her crying while bathing, praying to God to help her. She cried from a broken heart when she heard her daddy was having major surgery.

240

I begin to stir because I know she needs me. She has fallen onto the floor while trying to pull herself onto her wheelchair I think. She is frustrated and afraid to wake me so she is crying. I am so sound asleep that I can barely move my body. It seems to take forever before I can move my feet to touch the floor.

As I begin to swing my body around to the side of the bed I notice something is different. There is more than one voice. I hear something that I have heard before that has always cut to the quick of my heart. It is my children and they are weeping. I am overwhelmed with fear because this is more serious than I had imagined.

Standing up I head toward the family room and walking through the doorway I see my two boys holding onto their mother. She is crying. She is standing. Karen and my sons are walking toward me. I am overcome with emotion. "Praise God!" I exclaim. "He has answered our prayers!" With almost a giant leap toward them we embrace. "It's a miracle!" We exclaim.

Talking in rapid fashion Karen proclaims, "I just got up to use the bathroom and suddenly there was strength in my legs. They felt like they had not felt in a long time. I remembered that wonderful feeling and they were able to propel me up!"

Never has there been such rejoicing. Never has there been such hugging. "God thank you for being so good to us. Thank you for letting Karen walk again!"

It is a sweet time of prayer and giving God thanks. The night goes on for hours because there is so much joy in our house that we could never sleep. There are people to call.

There are Karen's parents. "Mom, Dad, I can walk!"

There are my parents. "Mom, Dad! Guess what is going on!"

"Son, we don't care it's two o'clock in the morning!"

"Dad get Mom on the phone I want to tell you something."

"Son this had better be good."

"It is good! Mom, Dad, Karen is walking again. We don't care that it's two in the morning. This is a miracle!"

I call my fellow church members. They have prayed for so long. They have been so faithful. I want them to know that God has answered their prayers and to know afresh and anew what a great God we serve. There is no end to the celebration. I am wired, as I have never been in my life.

"Come on Karen. Come on Jared and Zachary. Let's get into the car. We are going out!" We can't contain our excitement. There is this friend and then another one that we have to show what God has done.

Finally the night is catching up with us and we head back to our house.

"Dad we are so tired, but we are going to school tomorrow. We can't wait to tell our friends about what happened."

We kiss the boys goodnight. We look into the family room and there is the wheelchair. I walk over and fold it together and place it in our garage. The covers and sheets are removed from the couch.

I put my arms around Karen and I kiss her for the first time since I can't remember with her standing and her arms around me. Like always she is standing on her toes as she embraces me and I embrace her. Again for the first time since we can't remember we go to bed together.

Eventually I fall off to sleep. It is the kind of sleep I have not experienced in a long time. It is peaceful sleep. Suddenly there are no worries. It is such a wonderful feeling of contentment. I am where I am supposed to be--by Karen. And she is where she is supposed to be--beside me, embraced by my arms.

The sleep is blissful. It is unlike I have rested really ever before. For the first time I know what real peace is. My life is restored and everything is all right. It is more than all right. It is all I hoped it would ever be--again.

243

The morning comes and I awaken, my heart filled with the peace of delight. The smile across my face is surely a mile wide.

I turn over to reach for Karen. I must have rolled over and let go of Karen and I want to feel her in my arms once again and see the glow on her face because of her new and wonderful healthy body that has been restored. I discover she is gone. She must have gotten up to help the boys get off to school. That would be like her to get up and get them ready, fix their breakfast and never wake me.

I stumble into the kitchen. My face and heart falls. Something is wrong. There is Karen on the sofa. She is barely covered by a quilt. Her wheelchair is beside her.

I look up at the clock. It is only three in the morning. It has been a dream. It all has been one big dream. I walk into the boys' bedroom and Jared and Zachary are still asleep. They sleep so soundly they are almost it seems unconscious.

I walk back over to the couch where Karen is asleep. I pull the quilt and blanket up over her. She never moves.

Lying back down I struggle to go back to sleep. It was such a wonderful dream. I try to recapture what I had been dreaming, hoping that somehow I might once again enjoy the blissfulness of the moment.

But there is something happening to me. The surroundings of my three-bedroom house are suddenly transformed into the most glorious of splendors.

I have never seen anything like it. It is indescribable. The houses are the most beautiful houses I have ever seen. The yards are adorned with flowers. The trees have a look of springtime about them. There are waterfalls and brooks and small crystal clear streams flowing in and around the city.

The water is pure. The air is clean. There is an abundance of beauty and exquisite architecture. Some of the walls and buildings are made of beautiful stone. This city is so warm and inviting. There are smiling friendly people everywhere.

Two men with glowing faces greet me. They are beautiful and pure. They embrace me and with a smile lead me along the walkway. One says to me, "We are so glad you are here, Glenn." The other remarks, "There is nothing or no place like this."

They lead me to a special house that is unlike all of the others. There are Angels and Cherubim surrounding this house. Entering, my feet feel a little unsteady. I haven't felt this way since arriving here. I am nervous. And then I behold a man, with gentle eyes and a kind face. His gaze alone soothes my anxiety. His one look tells me all is all right.

There is a woman at His feet on her knees. She is worshipping Him. She adores and loves this man. The man extends His hand to her and in the same gesture He stretches His other hand toward me.

As He does I notice a rough looking scar in His hand that is palm up gesturing in my direction. The other hand, which has the hand of this young woman, is also palm up with her small hand barely in His and slightly covering another cruel scar. I look at these scars and seeing the countenance of His face I know without introduction whose presence I am in. And with almost the same breath I look into the face of Karen as she is fully standing. As she walks toward me with the strength of new legs. I cannot keep from crying. I am overwhelmed with joy for where I am and for where she is. Then suddenly this gentle hand that was holding hers moves toward my face and this wonderful man with the nail prints in His hands gently wipes the tears from my eyes.

With a very calm and assuring voice He said, "The journey you walked and lived is over. There will be none of what you experienced on earth here in this land. This is my Father's world. Come and let me show you the place I have prepared for you.

"Welcome," He said, "Into the joy of your Lord."

Chapter 39

From 1998 to November 2000

I finished the first of this manuscript in June of 1998. I understood things could and would likely become worse and they did.

We rented a hospital bed for Karen in the summer of 1999. For a period of time this bed was stationed in the family room because it enabled Karen to remain a part of the family hub of activities. A few months later we moved the bed into our bedroom because the time came when she would need attention during the night. At this current writing Karen cannot turn herself over in bed and this requires me to get up two and three times a night to turn her over.

Tremors began in March 2000 and have increased to where Karen can no longer feed herself. The best she can do is hold onto a bagel but with great difficulty. I feed her and hold her drink cups for her as she sips through a straw. Her hands began to tremor at first but now it is affecting her arms and head. So far the doctors have found nothing that can stop them. We are amazed that drugs are available that help persons with Parkinson's with their "shakes," but nothing yet has worked for Karen. This has been of all things so far the very most frustrating to her. No longer can she put her makeup on, brush her hair. Even handling the telephone and television remote has become almost impossible.

She has now moved to a special electric chair. We are grateful that Medicare made this possible. The cost of the chair was approximately $10,000 and would have been impossible for us. Her hands tremble so bad that she is barely able to use the hand control to maneuver the chair, yet the chair will transform to different positions enabling her body to adjust and have some comfort. It is a tremendous help.

Karen has to be lifted for everything that she does. She has no strength in her legs. Daily I lift her out of her bed at night. She has become a total invalid. Her legs and feet draw up toward her hips when I place her in bed. Many times I will try to stretch and manipulate them to give her a few minutes of rest. These moments of exercising her legs are a tremendous relief--briefly.

In May of this year I came home and found Jared and Zachary on their knees in front of their mother. She was sitting in a lazy boy chair in our bedroom. One of our caregivers had enabled her to sit there before leaving to go home. It was customary at that time for Karen to sit in this chair a couple of hours each day and watch television. Karen had managed to hide several bottles of pills underneath her quilt and overdosed after the lady left the house.

We called 911 and after four days in Intensive Care, Karen came through the suicide attempt. I never dreamed she would attempt it. When she came to and told me what she had done I was overwhelmed with emotion. Up until then I thought maybe she had accidentally taken a "few too many." I felt like my world had come to an end. I felt so bad because Karen felt this was her only option.

Later Karen would talk with regret that her attempt had not been successful. "Glenn, that was my only way out. I don't want to deal with this disease any longer. I don't want to end up in a nursing home. I know where all this is leading me. I want out before it gets to that point."

For six weeks Karen was in the hospital and then in a rehabilitation center. The people there were great to her and were the ones who eventually helped us obtain the wheelchair and even a free year's supply of Copaxone, which seems to be the most beneficial drug for Karen even though it has never turned her disease around. None of the drugs so far have purported to turn MS around, but only to slow down the progression of the disease.

After her suicide attempt Karen's neurologist put her on Lorazepam, a generic name for Ativan. This is a nerve pill that she started out taking three times a day and then eventually twice a day. This nerve pill became the greatest of all her medications as far as helping Karen's mental and emotional outlook. Karen was a beautifully sweet girl until MS and many of the negative medications took their toll on her. Lorazepam restored that beautiful sweetness. Unfortunately it was not until May of 1999 that Karen was put on any kind of nerve medication. This has been one of the greatest tragedies of all. She and our family had to deal with the mental nervous disorder caused by MS for ten years. It is unbelievable to me that with all the doctors we visited that somebody did not take the time to prescribe something that would stabilize Karen's emotions. When a person's entire body is shutting down and they are losing everything around them it only makes sense that some type of nerve medication has to be a vital daily essential.

So far nothing has slowed the progression of Karen's MS. Currently she is so weak I have to hold the telephone for her to have a conversation with her family in Ohio.

After returning home approximately ten women from our church have taken turns of coming to our house every day Monday through Friday. I had begun allowing them to come to our home only a couple of months before Karen's attempted suicide in the early spring. They had said for so long," We want to help." They have exercised Karen's legs and arms. They have fed her. They have done her hair and entertained her. They have done laundry and washed dishes and have been God's ministering angels to a struggling family trying to maintain some semblance of life. For them the Mollette family will always be grateful.

As of today, November 7, 2000 Karen has been back in the hospital for two weeks. Jared is now 18 and a high school senior. Zachary is 15 and a high school freshman. We literally hung our heads in sorrow a few nights ago as we made a decision to not allow the hospital to put a feeding tube in their mother's stomach. However, she has rallied and eating on her own once again.

I am in the position now of doing something I have never wanted to do—find a nursing home for Karen. There are nursing homes on every corner and I see few if any of them as being satisfactory for Karen. As she is in the hospital again at this moment I have no idea for sure if she will have to be placed in a nursing home or if I will be bringing her back home. I do not know if coming home is the best for her. Her need for care has become almost twenty-four hours. I do not know if it is best for our children. I do not know if it is best for me. However, having her home is easier than trying to go to the hospital every day.

The house is now incredibly lonely. I awake at 2:30 in the morning almost expecting to hear Karen say in the nicest way that she knows how to ask, "Glenn, do you mind helping me turn over, please?"

I at this moment am not quite for sure exactly what this illness is going to require of Karen before it takes her life. I do have fears about what she may have to face. I have no clue the kind of emotions that it is going to continue to drain out of my children and me. The grief and guilt that I sometimes feel for her being so sick at such a young age and for her maybe being placed in a nursing home are almost more than I can bear.

When this story ever really ends is in God's hands.

Author's note

Silent Struggler is my story of being a caregiver. To understand more about multiple sclerosis I would suggest you go to your local library and check out books on the subject. The average bookstore will have books about this and other diseases. Plus I invite you to read the stories of other caregivers and how they cared for their loved ones.

Multiple sclerosis now affects more than a half million people in the United States alone. There is no known cure for multiple sclerosis.

Printed in the United States
119601LV00002B/346/A

HELPING
CHRISTIANS
UNDERSTAND
Islam

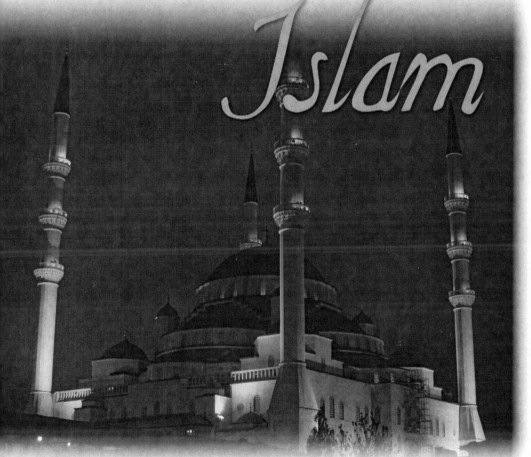

GEORGE AINSWORTH

ANM
publishers

Helping Christians Understand Islam

ISBN: 978-0-9715346-6-7 Paperback

Published by:

ANM
publishers

Advancing Native Missions
P.O. Box 5303
Charlottesville, VA 22905
www.adnamis.org

Acknowledgments

The author wishes to express his deep gratitude to all those whose support, encouragement, and prayers contributed to making this book a reality.

Thanks to those who helped in reading and editing. Special thanks to the leadership of ANM for their encouragement and direction, and for making this book's publication a practical reality.

Most of all, thanks to my dear wife of 34 years for her companionship in the adventure of following Jesus.

Table of Contents

Introduction   *Begin Here* 1

Chapter 1   *We Must Do Better* 5

Chapter 2   *God, Jesus, and the Scriptures* 23

Chapter 3   *Jews and Christians in Political Islam* 43

Chapter 4   *The Submission of* Dhimmis *and Slaves* 63

Chapter 5   *Ethics and Women* 81

Chapter 6   *Islam's Road to Triumph.* 99

Concluding Thoughts 121

Appendix I   *Muslim Jihad in Christian Ethiopia:*
Lessons for the West 127

Appendix II   Women in Osama Bin Laden's Thinking 131

Resources for Further Study 135

Introduction
Begin Here

Truth can be painful. This book sets forth the simple facts about what the sacred texts of Islam teach. The Koran, the Hadith (Mohammed's sayings), and the Sira (Mohammed's biography) are the basis for all Islamic law and practice. Many of these facts are not pleasant to learn, because they break down our preconceived notions of what "religion" is about. Many of these facts are not known even to Muslims, because most Muslims in the world do not speak or read Arabic. This is one of the reasons why many Muslims are quite friendly to non-Muslims.

This is a book for Christians. ANM's interaction with many Christian individuals and with congregations representing many different streams of Christianity has convinced us that Christians know very little about Islam. The popular media are not much help, for they either give us the reassuring line that "Islam is a religion of peace," or seek to incite us to anger by the latest act of Islamic terrorism.

We Christians are called to love Muslims, not hate them nor seek to harm them. On the other hand, when we approach Muslims to befriend them, it helps to know at least the basics of what Islam teaches, and the basics of what Muslims think Christians believe. It helps to know

1

where we have common ground and where we disagree. For example, Muslims and Christians are both monotheists. That is, both believe in one Supreme God. But Muslims often think that because Christians believe God is a Trinity that this means Christians are polytheists. It also helps to know that when Muslims and Christians use the same terms they mean something quite different by them, such as God being "merciful" and "compassionate." It also helps us as Christians to be clear what we believe so we speak what is true according to Scripture, and so we are better able to explain our faith to anyone, Muslim or otherwise, who wants to know about it.

Learning how to relate to Muslims in love is not complicated. As mentioned, a great many Muslims know only a part of what Islam teaches. For most Muslims, this is mostly the "religious" part of Islam. That is, what religious practices are commanded of Muslims, and what the Koran says about a Muslim's eternal destiny. It comes as a surprise even to many Muslims to learn that most of Islam's sacred texts are concerned with what Christians would call "political" questions. That is because Islam is a complete system of thought and behavior. It dictates what is to be done in every aspect of one's life in order to fully submit to God. "Islam" means "submission."

This book will help you as a Christian be clear about what you believe. It will also help you to understand why so many Muslims are quite nice people and why at the same time many are turning to acts of violence. Reading this book will give you some basic skills in answering questions Muslims may have about your faith, and also give you some questions to ask them, if they are open to discussion at all. It will help you understand why Islam is "another gospel" (Galatians 1:6-9), but also the many ways in which the Gospel of Christ is far more appealing than the revelation proclaimed by Mohammed. It will leave you rejoicing in your faith, and burdened to pray for those living in darkness. "The god of this world has blinded the minds of the unbelievers, to keep them from seeing the light of the gospel of the glory of Christ, who is the image of God" (II Corinthians 4:4).

Just a note, before we begin, on the spelling of Arabic words. Arabic words are written in Arabic script, not the "Latin" alphabet which is used for English. This means that an Arabic word must be transliterated to be used in English. In this book, for example, the name of the prophet of Islam is spelled "Mohammed." If you see it elsewhere spelled "Muhammad," it is the same name. Likewise for the Koran, which is often spelled "Qu'ran," when rendered in English. "Sura" in reference to the Koran, is equivalent to "Chapter." Chapters of the Koran are referred to by numbers and also by their titles.

The name of God revealed to Moses (Exodus 3:15) is indicated in the Hebrew original of the Old Testament by the Hebrew letters for YHWH. Modern scholars render this as "Yahweh." This rendering of God's Holy Name will be used in this book when it is necessary to distinguish God as He is revealed in the Bible from Allah who is proclaimed by Mohammed.

Finally, we at ANM would like to express our appreciation to Bill Warner, who has done great work in delineating the framework of what is political in Islam and distinguishing it from what is purely religious. He has also pioneered the helpful practice of analyzing the Islamic texts statistically to clarify what teachings are most important in Islam. Some of his books and his website www.politicalislam.com are referenced in the text and listed in the Resources for Further Study at the end of this book.

QUESTIONS:

1) Look through the book at the subheadings throughout each chapter. Which one are you most curious about?
2) Father, Son, and Holy Spirit appear in Mark 1:9-11. Is this a story of action by one God or three gods? Why?

Chapter 1
We Must Do Better

We Must Do Better Than This

[1] Two days after 9/11, the phone calls started going out to many churches. "Let us send a Muslim to your church and he will tell you about Islam, the peaceful religion." One church decided to go that one better. They invited a group of imams (the imams are Muslim religious leaders) and they also invited several Christian ministers. The Christians arrived that night in ones and twos. Then about the time the meeting was to start, in came all the Muslims. The imams came in as a group onto the stage and the Muslim men filed in next. They surrounded the Christians in their seats. And then the Muslim women came in all dressed in black from head to toe, and they sat in the back of the room. As Muslim women, they knew what their place was in public gatherings.

The first thing that happened was that an imam walked up to the lectern and placed a very large Koran on top and opened it up about half way. This was a symbolic act that was indicative of the entire night. The Christians didn't think anything about it one way or the other, but for the Muslims, it was a mark of whom they were and why they had come.

You see, Islam is a word that means submission. This word submission has several meanings. For the Muslim it means to submit to the Koran, the will of Allah and the sunna (THE WAY, THE EXAMPLE) of Mohammed. And all Muslims are required to make all others who are not Muslims submit to the Koran, to Allah, and to the sunna of Mohammed. They were there to dominate. What the Muslims did was to place the Koran as the focal point of dominance because this is where normally the Bible would have been. This act of dominance was symbolic of the night.

One of the imams got up and started to give his talk. He first said that Christians and Muslims worship the same God. Well, that seemed like a good foot to get started on. Since the Christians did not know anything about the character of Allah in the Koran that seemed fine to them. The imam went ahead and said they too honor Jesus because Jesus was a Muslim and a prophet of Allah. He also explained that Jesus was not the son of God, but merely a Muslim Prophet. And for that matter, the apostles were also Muslims. This came perhaps as a surprise to the Christians but they didn't say anything. The imam then went ahead to say that Jesus was not crucified, therefore was not resurrected. Muslims know this because this is what the Koran teaches.

The next thing the imam told the Christians was that the concept of the Trinity was a great affront to Allah. There is no such thing as the Trinity, and believing it makes Christians polytheists. The fact that the Christians are viewed as polytheists explains something that happened at the beginning when the minister first said "Let us pray together." There was almost a panicked response from the imams at this. "No," they said, "No! We do not pray with others." This was quite puzzling to the Christian minister but since the Christians were there as hosts and they were there to be kind and polite, he didn't say anything. But not knowing anything about Islam, you could tell from the puzzled look on the minister's face that he was thinking, "Why would they object to praying together?" The reason is that the Christians are viewed as polytheists. To pray with them is a terrible sin, so terrible that it has a special name, shirk. The Koran says that if they had prayed with the Christians, they would definitely go to hell. Praying with the Christians would have been a sin worse than mass murder, because murder can be excused under the proper circumstances, but praying with polytheists cannot. By the way, Muslims typically think the Christian Trinity is 3 gods: God, Jesus, and Mary, so Christians are polytheists.

Again the Christians did not understand anything about Islam or they would have never made the invitation to prayer. Or they would have simply prayed while the Muslims sat there. The Muslims dominated on this point. There, inside a Christian Church as guests, there would be no prayers with the Christians.

Another thing that the imam said in his talk was that the New Testament was a corrupt document and was in error. Not only was the New Testament in error, so was the Old Testament. In particular, the reason that the New Testament was wrong was that Jesus' chief prophecy was left out of it. That prophecy, according to the Koran, was that after Jesus the final prophet would come and his name would be Ahmed. (Ahmed and Mohammed are two forms of the same name, like Bill and William). The imam said Christians had removed these prophecies from the New Testament. This was one of the many reasons that the New Testament was a document which was simply wrong. If Christians wanted to learn the real story of Jesus what they would have to do is to read the Koran because the Koran contains the exact truth about Isa, the Arabic word for Jesus.

Imagine if the Christian minister had stood up and made assertions such as that Mohammed was not a prophet of any sort, that the Koran was a derivative work, that it is was just a book in which things were copied from the Jews and Christians, Zoroastrians and the old Arabic religions, that Allah was simply the tribal moon god of the Korash (or Quraish) tribe. That would have been equivalent to what the Muslim imam said but the Christians didn't do that for two reasons. One, they were the hosts and they were going to be polite. The other reason was they knew nothing about the Koran. In response to questions from the audience, none of the Christians had read the Koran nor had they read the traditions of Mohammed, the Hadith. Nor did they know anything about Mohammed's life. But the imams had read the New Testament and the Old Testament. So they knew about the Christians while the Christians knew nothing about them. This was the way the entire night went. The Christians were asked questions by the Muslims and the questions the Muslims asked were 1400 years old. These were stock questions but the Christians were caught flat-footed. They had never thought about these kinds of questions before. The Muslims came prepared and the Christians were not prepared. In this book you will learn information to help you deal with common Muslim approaches when speaking with non-Muslims, and how to better explain your Christian faith to Muslims.

The ministers present admitted they didn't know anything about the history of Christianity and Islam. This is tragic, dreadfully tragic, because over 60 million Christians and over 210 million other people: Africans, Hindus, Buddhists, and others, have been killed in the process of the purposeful expansion of Islam known as jihad. How did Turkey, which is 99.7 percent Islamic, go from a Greek Christianized culture, to being Islamic? The Christians in the church that night didn't know how this process happened. They also didn't know that in the 20th century alone some 1.5 million Armenians who belonged to the Armenian Orthodox Church were killed in Turkey. Why didn't the ministers know these dreadful facts? Very simply, it's because although they went to divinity school, no one ever mentioned it. They had never been taught the history or doctrine of Islam. They didn't know, for instance, that most Islamic teaching deals with what we would call political ideology, not religion. But then, to devout Muslims, there is no difference between the two. To submit to Allah as he is revealed by his prophet Mohammed means that all of life: personal, cultural, political, and economic, is to be governed by what Allah has declared.

Basics

As a starting point, let us compare two classic simple statements of faith. The first is basic to both Judaism and Christianity:

"**Hear O Israel, the LORD (Yahweh) our God, the LORD
(Yahweh) is One, and you shall love the LORD (Yahweh)**

your God with all your heart and with all your soul and with all your strength." Deuteronomy 6:4

Then there is this statement, the entry point to Islam.

"There is one God, Allah, and Mohammed is the prophet of Allah." This is the *shahada*, or basic Muslim confession of faith. Reciting this simple statement in Arabic before Muslims makes you a Muslim. "Islam" means "submission." A "Muslim" is a person who has submitted.

The obvious similarity between these two confessions of faith is that God is One. The obvious contrast is between the command to love profoundly on the one hand versus asserting the supremacy of Mohammed on the other. To make this even clearer by turning it around, the Bible does NOT say: "There is one God, Yahweh, and Moses is his prophet," On the other hand, while there are a few Koranic injunctions to love Allah by obeying him, these are peripheral, not central. Obedience is central, while "love," in the sense of Deuteronomy 6:4, is not. There is more on this in the next chapter.

The Source of Muslim teaching

"Mohammed is the prophet of Allah" means that: 1) everything Mohammed said or did declares what Islam is, and 2) everything Mohammed said or did takes precedence over what any other prophet ever said or did. Therefore:

1a) The Koran contains what Mohammed said the angel Gabriel said that Allah said. Mohammed's companions could not hear anything. Only Mohammed ever claimed to hear what Gabriel was saying. Mohammed claimed that the Koran was exactly what Allah had dictated. The Koran is the literal words of Allah because Mohammed said so. The Koran is believed by Muslims to be Allah's literal word-for-word dictation in Arabic to Mohammed via Gabriel. Therefore the actual Koran only exists in Arabic. Any translation is automatically an interpretation of the actual Koran, not the Koran itself.

1b) The next important source for Islamic doctrine is the Hadith. These are sayings of Mohammed repeated by his companions and later recorded. The Muslim scholar Bukhari, whose collection of these sayings is considered the most authoritative, compiled them from both written and oral sources over a 16 year period ending in 846 AD. The other most authoritative collection, that of al-Muslim, was compiled some time between 834-895 AD. In both cases we are looking at a time period some 200 years after the death of Mohammed.

1c) The other source of Muslim doctrine is Sira, the biography of Mohammed. The most authoritative is by Ibn Ishaq, His date of birth is obscure, perhaps 704 AD, but he is known to have died about 140 years after Mohammed, so he wrote his biography more than 100 years after Mohammed's death.

The Hadith and Sira together make up "Sunna," the life and traditions about Mohammed. All Islamic teaching must be based on the Koran and Sunna.

2a) The Koran mentions a number of previous prophets of Allah, including Adam, Noah, Abraham, Moses, David, and Jesus. However, it declares that Mohammed's revelation is superior to, and supersedes, that which Allah gave to them.

2b) When the Koran describes the message of any of these earlier prophets of Allah, those familiar with the Bible will immediately see differences in the story. For example, in the Koran the reason Pharaoh is punished with plagues is not because he will not let the Hebrews go, but because he does not recognize that Moses is a prophet of Allah. In the case of Jesus, the Koran does not describe Jesus as dying for our sins, nor does it mention him proclaiming the Kingdom of God. Instead, it declares that Jesus' purpose as a prophet was to announce the future coming of Mohammed.

2c) When dealing with the discrepancy between the Bible's presentation of people and events and the Koran's presentation, Islam's explanation is clear. The Jews and Christians have corrupted their Scriptures. That is why they no longer speak what is true about the earlier prophets. But Allah, by Mohammed, has revealed everything correctly.

The Source of Christian teaching

The Christian Bible contains 66 books written over more than 1500 years by at least 40 different authors in 3 different languages. Although the original writers were inspired by God, and guided by Him in what they wrote (II Timothy 3:16; II Peter 1:21), the Bible's meaning can be understood in any language when properly translated. Despite the diversity of times, background, and language, the entire Bible contains a unity of theme which we often summarize as the "Gospel", or "Good News." This unity emerges clearly in the teaching of Jesus himself. "Beginning with Moses and all the Prophets, he (Jesus) interpreted to them in all the Scriptures the things concerning himself" (Luke 24:27). In other words, the central message of the Christian Bible is about Jesus: who He is, why He came, how we are to respond to Him. The Bible presents our response to Him as the key to human life now and forever. "There is salvation in no one else, for there is no other name (than Jesus) under heaven given among men by which we must be saved" (the apostle Peter in Acts 4:12). "Who is the liar but he who denies that Jesus is the Christ? This is the antichrist, who denies the Father and the Son. No one who denies the Son has the Father. Whoever confesses the Son has the Father also." (the apostle John in I John 2:22-23). "Even if we or an angel from heaven should preach to you a gospel contrary to the one we preached to you, let him be accursed" (the apostle Paul in Galatians 1:8). Or in the famous words of Jesus Himself: "I am the way, the truth, and the life. No one comes to the Father except through me" (Gospel of John 14:6).

The source of Christian teaching is the Bible as it presents Jesus Christ who is the center of God's plan for the human race. We can summarize the Gospel, this "Master Plan" this way:

1) God created everything in the universe good. He created human beings good, and in His very image, capable of relationship with Him and of acting as His vice regents in governing Creation.

2) The human race from the beginning disobeyed God and fell out of relationship with Him. Through the Fall, human beings lost the gift of eternal life and their authority over Creation.

3) God came as a man, Jesus, to complete the work of restoring the human race to relationship with Himself, and to restore it to His intended place of authority in the universe. Jesus did this by living a life without sin, then offering His life on the cross to take the rightful punishment for our sin in our place. He rose from the dead and assumed authority over the created Universe.

4) All those who put their faith in Jesus and what He has done have forgiveness of sins, receive the gift of eternal life, and are restored to God's original created purpose for the human race. The present age exists for the primary purpose of bringing those from every part of the human family into this family of those who have been restored to God through Jesus Christ. This is done by proclaiming who Jesus is and what He has done. All who choose to put their trust in Him become Christians.

5) The consummation of this process will be the return of Jesus in visible triumph over all things, including over all those who refused to believe in Him.

You will notice that the Gospel includes nothing that can be called political, as such, during this present age. There are certainly political implications in such doctrines as "every person is created in the image of God," but there is not a specific political program such as that laid down in the Koran, Hadith, and Sira. Islam as practiced by many, probably the majority, of Muslims is primarily religious. Practicing Muslims follow the "Five Pillars:" reciting the creed (the *shahada*), praying five times daily while facing Mecca, fasting during Ramadan, giving to Muslim charities, and making a pilgrimage to Mecca. But most of the Islamic doctrine taught by Mohammed is primarily what we would call a political ideology.

Mohammed

Islam is based entirely upon Mohammed. The way to know Islam is to know Mohammed's life and words.[2] Mohammed was born in Mecca about 570 AD. At about age 40 he started to have visions and hear voices which he initially feared were demonic, but which his wife convinced him to accept. The voices told him that he was the prophet of Allah. He began to tell others of his message, and that they should stop worshipping idols and worship Allah as the one God in the manner revealed to Mohammed. After about 13 years and a modest number of converts, the Meccans forced Mohammed to flee in 622 AD and he went to Medina. Once in Medina, Mohammed's voices taught him to be a politician and warlord. In Medina he developed the concept of jihad, sacred striving for Allah, with an emphasis on violent striviing. Over the next 10 years Mohammed crushed all his opponents on the Arabian peninsula and become ruler of Arabia. He died of an apparent illness in 632 AD. The Sira, the authorized biography of Mohammed, gives much detail about him, including his appearance, how he ate, his emotions, and his family life. The Koran says over 70 times that Muslims are to copy Mohammed's life in every detail.

When Mohammed's visions and voices began, he was about age 40. During the month of Ramadan, he was violently confronted (choked) by a being he later identified as the angel Gabriel. This being, while choking him, demanded he "Recite! Recite!" meaning "Say what you're told to say!" Once he had decided, because of his wife's endorsement, that his angelic encounter was from God, he began to declare (Recite!) the message as it came to him, often in poetry. Some of his early preaching included:

✦ Allah (which means "god" in Arabic) was not merely the moon god of the Meccans, he was the only true God

✦ Mohammed was Allah's prophet

✦ All who did not worship Allah as directed by Mohammed were going to Hell, and all the Meccans' dead ancestors were already in Hell. This was not popular, and was part of why Mohammed was eventually required to leave Mecca in 622 AD.

This leaving Mecca is known as the "*Hijra*," or "Immigration." It is so important that the Islamic calendar starts from this point.[3] The Islamic calendar does not date years as "A.D.", but as "A.H.", the year of the Hijra. The first year in Medina, Mohammed and the Muslims who went with him were very poor. Allah told Mohammed to raid the caravans of those who did not believe in his message. These raids failed seven times, but succeeded on the eighth time. From then on, Mohammed was successful, and, as his number of followers increased, he went from caravan raiding to open war against first the Meccans and then the Jews of Medina and the nearby region. In the Koran, Mohammed is urged to warfare, jihad, against those who do not accept Allah as their one true God and Mohammed as his prophet. Some Jews who were not annihilated were, at Allah's direction, made into a new category of semi-slave known as a *dhimmi*. Mohammed was consistently ruthless in killing all who had openly opposed him. For example, when he conquered Mecca, his home town, he executed two dancing girls who had sung a satirical song about him. One of his previous secretaries had fled Medina for Mecca because he began to suspect that Mohammed was making up his revelations. This man was executed as well. Mohammed's dying words were a command that no Jews or Christians were to remain in Arabia, only Muslims.

When Mohammed died, he had appointed no successor, so Abu Bakr, Mohammed's closest companion, was chosen as leader, or "Caliph." Now that Mohammed was gone, many tried to leave Islam, so Abu Bakr spent the two years of his caliphate killing all who tried. After he died a natural death, another companion of Mohammed, Umar, became Caliph. Umar spent 10 years in jihad against mainly-Christian Egypt, Syria, Iraq, and Persia. A Persian he had enslaved then killed Umar. The next caliph was Uthman, another companion of Mohammed. He ruled 12 years, then was killed by Abu Bakr's grandson in a political dispute. After him was Ali, Mohammed's son-in-law. He was implicated in the plot that killed Uthman, and Aisha, Mohammed's favorite wife, led a war against Ali in which he and his two sons were killed. The killing of Ali and his sons is the origin of the division between Shia Muslims (supporters of Ali) and Sunni Muslims, who are the majority. So Mohammed's family and closest followers, those who knew him best, unhesitatingly followed his example of ruthlessness. Jihad, violence to advance the cause of Allah and force submission, was commanded in the Koran and demonstrated by Mohammed's example. Unfortunately, this means that the 9/11 attackers were not acting in a non-Islamic manner, but following the example of Mohammed. It is possible for Muslims to deny this, however, as Muslim spokesmen often do. We will look at why this is possible, but first we need to clarify the concept of Jihad.

Jihad

"Jihad" means "struggle." It does not necessarily mean killing. It means the struggle on behalf of Allah against all that resists him. It includes the struggle against one's own non-Islamic tendencies, but only 3% of the jihad Hadith refer to this. The overwhelming majority of texts about jihad, which include 24% of the entire Koran from the Medina period, 21% of all the Hadith, and 67% of the Sira, Mohammed's life, deal with jihad against non-Muslims, for whom there is a special denigrating term: *kafir*. So all struggle to bring *kafirs* into submission to Islam is jihad. This means that building a mosque is jihad.[4] Writing a pro-Islam letter to the editor is jihad. Marrying a non-Muslim woman so that all the children are raised as Muslims is jihad. Enslaving *kafir* populations is jihad.

Sometimes people learn of the violence associated with Islam and say: "Yes, but God in the Old Testament commands violence, too." No doubt about it, but in the Old Testament it is always violence against a particular group of people who were endangering the people of God at a particular point in time. It is never made into a universal ethical and political doctrine. Only about 5.6% of the Old Testament text concerns acts of political violence, and in the New Testament, of course, violence on behalf of Christ is forbidden. "All who take the sword will perish by the sword" (Jesus in Matthew 26:52). When Christians in the Middle Ages decided to launch the Crusades, regardless of whether you think this was appropriate or not, they did not do so because it was commanded in Holy Scripture, but in response to four and a half centuries of anti-

Christian jihad by the followers of Mohammed. Mohammed became successful when he made political violence a part of Islam. So, in contrast to the 5.6% of the text of the Old Testament that concerns acts of political violence, about 31% of the sacred texts of Islam are concerned with political violence. 67% of the Sira, the authoritative biography of Mohammed, describes his acts of political violence, about one every six weeks for the last nine years of his life.[5]

Dualism, or duality, in Islam

Bill Warner in his <u>Thirteen Talks on Political Islam</u> helpfully delineates how often in Islam there are two aspects to things.

Every person is either a Muslim or a kafir. All Muslims belong to the House of Islam. All *kafirs* belong to the House of War. It is every Muslim's duty to bring everyone into the House of Islam by whatever means necessary.

There are two Mohammeds. The early Mohammed in Mecca was a preacher who condemned idolatry and called people to worship one true God. The early Mohammed threatened unbelievers with Hell in the afterlife. The message of the early Mohammed was religious in nature. The early Mohammed was not very successful. He attracted perhaps 150 followers and was forced out of his home town. The later Mohammed was a warlord and political leader. He used the doctrine of jihad to promote Muslims assassinating, robbing, and making war. He threatened unbelievers with death, slavery, and political oppression. The message of the later Mohammed was political in nature. The later Mohammed was extremely successful. In 10 years he became sole ruler of all Arabia.

In the same way, in parallel with Mohammed's life, **there are effectively two Korans.**[6] In the Koran, chapters (Sura) are arranged by length, not by when Mohammed received them. However, scholars have reconstructed which sayings go with which parts of Mohammed's life. The Meccan Koran says nothing about Jihad and only 1% of its verses are anti-Jewish. Most references to Jews and Christians are positive. For example, Christians are encouraged to take heed to the scriptures they have so they will be able to stand in the Day of Judgment. But in the Medinan Koran 24% of the verses are about Jihad. Seventeen percent of it is anti-Jewish. By comparison, only 7% of the text of Hitler's <u>Mein Kampf</u> (which, interestingly enough, means "My Struggle"), is anti-Jewish. It is in the Medinan Koran where we find Christians also considered kafirs. *"Make war on those who have received the Scriptures (Jews and Christians) but do not believe in Allah or the Last Day. They do not forbid what Allah and His Messenger have forbidden. The Christians and Jews do not follow the religion of truth until they submit and pay the jizya (a special per-capita tax for kafirs), and they are humiliated"* (Sura 9:29 Yusuf Ali authorized translation).

The duality of the Koran shows clearly in a pair of texts like the following (Yusuf Ali's authorized translation):

> From the Meccan Koran: *"Listen to what they (unbelievers) say with patience, and leave them with dignity"* (73:10)
>
> From the Medinan Koran: *"Then your Lord spoke to His angels and said, 'I will be with you. Give strength to the believers (Muslims). I will send terror into the Kafirs' hearts, cut off their heads and even the tips of their fingers!"* (8:12).

This duality within the Koran itself, coupled with the fact that the majority of the world's Muslims do not speak or read Arabic, is one of the reasons why many Muslims simply go about their lives quietly, without any involvement in violent jihad. If they belong to a mosque whose imam preaches mainly out of the Meccan Koran, then their concept of Islam will be quite different than those exposed to the fullness of Mohammed's revelation.

Islamic ethics are also dualistic. There is one ethic for relationships among Muslims and another for relationships with non-Muslims, *kafirs*. A Muslim may deceive kafirs, especially if the purpose is to advance the cause of Islam. There is even a word for this sacred deception, *taqiyya*.

Most religions and ethical systems have some form of what we call "The Golden Rule." C.S. Lewis points this out in his section on *"The Tao"* in <u>The Abolition of Man</u>. Jesus' version of this is: **"whatever you wish that** others would do to you, do also to them, for this is the Law and the Prophets" (Matthew 7:12). Jesus told the parable of the Good Samaritan to emphasize that the command "love your neighbor as yourself" (Leviticus 19:18) is universal. But in Islam, only a fellow Muslim qualifies as a "neighbor." A *kafir* can never be a "neighbor" in that sense. Thus in George W. Bush's book about his presidency, <u>Decision Points</u>, he describes the surprise of an African Muslim woman when she is helped by a Catholic charity. In the same way, in the fascinating autobiography <u>A God Who Hates</u> by former Muslim Dr. Wafa Sultan, she describes her shock at the kindness shown her by a Jewish neighbor after she moved to America. Both these women were astonished because they were encountering the Golden Rule in operation for the first time.

Deception and Abrogation

In Islam, Allah himself uses deception to advance his cause.

> But they (the Jews) *were deceptive*, and Allah *was deceptive, for Allah is the best of deceivers* (*Wamakaroo wamakara Allahu waAllahu khayru al-makireena*)! Sura 3:54; cf. 8:30

> Are they then secure from *Allah's deception (makra Allahi)?* None deemeth himself secure from *Allah's deception (makra Allahi)* save folk that perish. Sura 7:99

> So they schemed a scheme: and We schemed a scheme (Wamakaroo makran wamakarna makran), while they perceived not. Sura 27:50

Obviously, if Allah uses deception, then it is proper to lie if it will advance the cause of Islam.

Also in Islam, it is accepted that the words of God are contradictory. Here is the example we looked at previously:

> *"Listen to what they (unbelievers) say with patience, and leave them with dignity"* (73:10) This sounds good, doesn't it?

HELPING CHRISTIANS UNDERSTAND *Islam*

"Then your Lord spoke to His angels and said, 'I will be with you. Give strength to the believers (Muslims). I will send terror into the Kafirs' hearts, cut off their heads and even the tips of their fingers!" (8:12). Not so good!

Because both statements are in the Koran, which Muslims believe has been dictated by Allah himself, both are true. So Muslims may use either in advancing the cause of Islam. But when Muslims must decide which text has absolute precedence, they apply another doctrine, the doctrine of abrogation. Abrogation means that Allah can, and does, cancel out things he has said previously by things he says later on.

> *Allah effaceth what He will, and establisheth (what He will), and with Him is the source of ordinance. (13:39, Pickthall's translation).*

> *And if We willed We could withdraw that which We have revealed unto thee, then wouldst thou find no guardian for thee against Us in respect thereof. (Pickthall, 17:86)*

> *Nothing of our revelation (even a single verse) do we abrogate or cause be forgotten, but we bring (in place) one better or the like thereof. Knowest thou not that Allah is Able to do all things? (Pickthall, 2:106)*

Therefore, later words of Allah take precedence over words he spoke earlier. For example, all the "friendly" verses about Jews and Christians which are part of the Meccan Koran are abrogated by the verses of the Medinan Koran which express hatred toward them. But since all the words of the Koran, even the abrogated ones, are the words of God, all of them can be used in the cause of advancing Islam. So when it is helpful to quote the friendly words about Jews and Christians, it is quite proper to do so.

Summing up:

Islam is not just a religion, nor just a system of conduct for individuals, but an ideology that prescribes what God demands in every aspect of political, social, cultural, and economic life.

The basis for what Islam requires is what is in the Koran (in which Mohammed recites the words he says he received from God through the angel Gabriel) plus Mohammed's sayings as recorded in the Hadith plus the example of Mohammed's life as recorded in the Sira, his biography. All Islamic law (*sharia*) is based upon these texts.

Therefore, it is not helpful to cite the example of particular Muslims, good or bad, in trying to establish what Islam is, any more than the example of particular Christians, good or bad, establishes what Christianity is.

Christians are those who put their faith in Jesus Christ and what He has done for us. That faith, if genuine, will produce lives that increasingly resemble the example of Jesus. So when the members of a Kansas church show up at military funerals and insult the dead and their families, we can say they are not acting like Christians.

On the other hand, a Muslim is one who follows the words and deeds of Mohammed. So when Muslims rioted and killed innocent *kafirs* in response to cartoons of Mohammed in a Danish newspaper, this was in accordance with Mohammed's own life and example. Mohammed was completely intolerant of every insult, and taught that all kafirs have committed the unforgiveable offense of denying that Mohammed is the prophet of the one true God. If Mohammed is not who he said he was, this means God is not as Mohammed describes him, and Islam is false. This thought is unspeakably offensive to Muslims. Nothing is too severe toward those who promote it or believe it.

In contrast, Jesus taught **"Blessed are you when others revile you and persecute you and utter all kinds of evil against you falsely on my account. Rejoice and be glad, for your reward is great in heaven."** (Matt. 5:11). He also taught: "if anyone slaps you on the right cheek, turn to him the other also . . . Love your enemies and pray for those who persecute you" (Matt. 5:39, 44).

Islam and Christianity present two very different views of what pleases God and how we should act toward other human beings. It's important for us, especially in these days, to decide what we believe and practice it.

QUESTIONS:

1. This chapter uses a simple 5-point framework to describe the Gospel message. What other points, if any, would you include in explaining the Gospel to someone?

2. Which contrasts between Christianity and Islam in this chapter stand out most clearly to you?

Endnotes:

1   Adapted from Bill Warner's _Thirteen Lessons on Political Islam_ Number 6 '"The Christians." May be downloaded from the Internet in its entirety at http://www.politicalislam.com/ blog/category/thirteen-talks-on-political-islam/

2   Read, for example, A Simple Koran or the condensed version An Abridged Koran. These correlate the Koranic revelations with events in Mohammed's life. http://www. cspipublishing.com

3   The importance of the _Hijra_ in connecting Muslim immigration and _jihad_ is examined in detail in Modern Day Trojan Horse: the Islamic Doctrine of Immigration by Sam Solomon & E. Almaqdisi. Pilcrow Press 2009.

4   The essential role of the mosque in encouraging all forms of jihad is dealt with in The Mosque Exposed by Sam Solomon & E. Almaqdisi. ANM Publishers 2006.

5   For the value of statistical analysis in studying Islam see Bill Warner http://www. politicalislam.com/blog/statistics-and-the-meaning-of-islam/.   Warner's detailed statistical analysis of Islamic texts can be found at http://www.politicalislam.com/ downloads/Statistical-Islam.pdf

6   This, again, is clearly seen by correlating Koranic texts with events in Mohammed's life, such as in An Abridged Koran: the Reconstructed Historical Koran Bill Warner, ed. CSPI Publishing 2006.

Chapter 2
God, Jesus, and the Scriptures

To review the previous chapter...

Islam is not just a religion, nor just a system of conduct for individuals, but an ideology that prescribes in detail what God demands in every aspect of political, social, cultural, and economic life.

The basis for what Islam requires is what is in the Koran (in which Mohammed recites the words he says he received from God through the angel Gabriel) plus Mohammed's sayings as recorded in the Hadith plus the example of Mohammed's life as recorded in the Sira, his biography. All Islamic law (sharia) is based upon these texts.

As pointed out in the previous chapter, Christians are those who put their faith in Jesus Christ and what He has done for us. Who Jesus is and what He has done for us is revealed in the Bible, including both the Old and New Testaments.

On the other hand, a Muslim is one who follows the words and deeds of Mohammed.

Islam and Christianity present two very different views of what pleases God and how we should act toward other human beings. That's why the previous chapter points out how important it is for us, especially in these days, to be clear what we believe and practice it. What we actually believe will influence what we do. Jesus put it this way:

Luke 6:43-45

"For no good tree bears bad fruit, nor again does a bad tree bear good fruit, for each tree is known by its own fruit. For figs are not gathered from thorn bushes, nor are grapes picked from a bramble bush. The good person out of the good treasure of his heart produces good, and the evil person out of his evil treasure produces evil, for out of the abundance of the heart his mouth speaks."

This chapter will examine ways in which Christianity and Islam teach both similar and very different things about God, about Jesus, about the best source of spiritual authority, about human nature, and about the way of salvation.

Who is God? What is God's nature?

One Chief Similarity

Islam and Christianity agree together on the existence of God, One Supreme Being, and disagree with any purely materialist worldview, whether ancient or modern. As C.S. Lewis puts it so well in his classic Mere Christianity:

> "Ever since men were able to think, they have been wondering what this universe really is and how it came to be there. And, very roughly, two views have been held. First, there is what is called the materialist view. People who take that view think that matter and space just happen to exist, and always have existed, nobody knows why; and that the matter, behaving in certain fixed ways, has just happened, by a sort of fluke, to produce creatures like ourselves who are able to think. By one chance in a thousand something hit our sun and made it produce

the planets; and by another thousandth chance the chemicals necessary for life, and the right temperature, occurred on one of these planets, and so some of the matter on this earth came alive; and then, by a very long series of chances, the living creatures developed into things like us. The other view is the religious view. According to it, what is behind the universe is more like a mind than it is like anything else we know."

Christianity and Islam agree that the physical universe is not all there is, and that the universe cannot account for its own existence. A Mind which exists apart from the universe has produced it. This fundamental agreement is reflected, for example, in one common approach taken by both Muslim Medieval philosophers and the great Medieval Christian philosopher Thomas Aquinas. Both adopted forms of the following argument for the existence of God. It is known as the Cosmological argument. It states:

Whatever begins to exist has a cause of its existence.

The universe began to exist.

Therefore, the universe has a cause of its existence.

God in both Christianity and Islam is identified as that uncaused cause of the universe. God is the Creator of all that is, apart from Himself. To the self-styled critic who says: "Oh yeah, well who caused God?" both Muslim and Christian thinkers over the centuries have pointed out that the question misses the point. God never began to exist, so the argument doesn't apply to Him.

Or, another way to answer the question "Who caused God?" is to say: "God did." "You mean God is the eternally sufficient cause of His own existence?" "That's right."

Disagreements

Having agreed that there is One God who is the Creator of the Universe, we immediately move into areas of outright disagreement, or of differences in emphasis that produce very different results.

For an example of outright disagreement, the Koran clearly says of Allah that Allah is deceptive, for *"Allah is the best of deceivers (Wamakaroo wamakara Allahu waAllahu khayru al-makireena)"*! S. 3:54

This produces the Islamic doctrine of *taqiyya*, namely, that to practice deception in the cause of Allah is no sin, since Allah himself practices deception in his own cause.

In sharp contrast, the Bible clearly says of Yahweh, the LORD:

Numbers 23:19

"God is not a man, that He should lie, nor a son of man, that He should repent; Has He said, and will He not do it? Or has He spoken, and will He not make it good?

1 Samuel 15:29

"Also the Glory of Israel will not lie or change His mind; for He is not a man that He should change His mind."

This produces the Biblical doctrine (for both Jews and Christians), that deception is morally wrong, especially if the intent is to cause harm to another human being. It is the integrity of God's own nature which He calls us to imitate in the 9th Commandment: "You shall not bear false witness against your neighbor."

In the Koran, it is an aspect of Allah's supremacy that he should be a far more clever deceiver than those who plot against him. In the Bible, it is an aspect of Yahweh's supremacy that integrity is part of His nature. Because He is truly Sovereign, he never needs to deceive in order to accomplish His purposes.

Now let's look at an example of where there is a similarity of terminology regarding who God is, but where the same term means something different.

In Christianity, LOVE is an essential part of who God is, His nature. "God is love" I John 4:8. Because God IS love, He is relational by nature, even within Himself. For example, Jesus calls God "Father" even while asserting that He and the Father are One, and then asserts that those who believe in Him will share in their unity. "Holy Father, keep them in your Name, which you have given me, that they may be one, even as we are one" (John 17:11). The love resident in the Godhead may be entered into by the believer. In Christianity, God IS knowable, even by puny and sinful human beings, because He has chosen to humble Himself, becoming incarnate as Jesus Christ and taking upon Himself the just punishment for our sins, so that we CAN know Him. Human beings were created for relationship with God, and can know God as well as be known by Him.

In Islam, who Allah is in himself is unknowable, as there is no one and nothing to which he can be compared. There is a term in Islam for this solitary incomparable oneness, *tawhid*. To associate anyone or anything with Allah, or even presume to describe what he is like in himself is impossible. Those who do so commit *shirk*, the worst possible sin.

Islam uses "99 names" to describe Allah, but these do not describe who He is in himself, but rather the kind of actions that result from His will. Most of these names declare his power and splendor, but some declare his mercy, compassion, and forgiveness. These are not considered part of Allah's nature as such, but rather actions which Allah is free to take or not to take. He is not merciful because he is loving in nature. He is merciful because he chooses to be, when he chooses to be. All of God's "names" in Islam are based on actions of his will. Because he sometimes chooses to be merciful or compassionate, he is called "Allah the merciful, the compassionate."

Therefore the "love" of Allah is a description of His attitudes and actions toward people. So the Koran teaches:

Allah loves those who are spiritual, pure and clean—al-Baqarah 2:222

Allah loves those who do good—al-Baqarah 2:195; Âl'Imran 3:134

Allah loves those who keep faith and act rightly—Âl'Imran 3:76

In all the examples above, the love of Allah is conditional upon the believer acting rightly. If the believer should turn back from Allah, Allah does not love him any more (Âl'Imran 3:32).

Allah emphatically does NOT love kafirs:

> "O ye who believe! Choose not My enemy and your enemy for allies. Do ye give them friendship when they disbelieve in that truth which hath come unto you, driving out the messenger and you because ye believe in Allah, your Lord? If ye have come forth to strive in My way and seeking My good pleasure, (show them not friendship). Do ye show friendship unto them in secret, when I am Best Aware of what ye hide and what ye proclaim? And whosoever doeth it among you, he verily hath strayed from the right way." (al-Mumtahanah 60:1 Pickthall's translation).

While there are over 300 references in the Koran to Allah and fear, there are 49 references to love. Of these love references, 39 are negative. There are 14 negative references to love of money, power, other gods and status, and there are 25 verses about how Allah does not love kafirs. Three verses command humanity to love Allah and two verses are about how Allah loves a believer. This leaves five verses about love. Of these five, three are about loving kin or a Muslim brother. One verse commands a Muslim to give for the love of Allah. This leaves only the verse that commands giving what you love to "charity," which always means charity toward other Muslims.

By contrast, the New Testament declares God's love toward everyone: "For God so loved the world that he gave his only begotten Son that whoever believes in him shall not perish, but have everlasting life" (John 3:16).

"The Lord is not slow to fulfill his promise, as some count slowness, but is patient toward you, not wishing that any should perish, but that all should reach repentance" (II Peter 3:9). Jesus bluntly says: "I did not come to call the righteous, but sinners" (Mark 2:17).

This aspect of God's attitude toward the disobedient and unbelieving is seen throughout the Old Testament as well. For example, in Hosea, Yahweh says: "How can I give you up, O Ephraim? How can I hand you over, O Israel? . . . My heart recoils within me; my compassion grows warm and tender. I will not execute my burning anger; I will not again destroy

Ephraim; for I am God and not a man, the Holy One in your midst, and I will not come in wrath" (Hosea 11:8-9).

Or consider the example of Jonah. The prophet was reluctant to preach to the Gentiles of Nineveh, people who did NOT worship the God of Israel, precisely because he knew God's compassionate nature. When Nineveh repents, God relents, saying to Jonah: *"You pity the plant, for which you did not labor, not did you make it grow . . . should I not pity Nineveh, that great city, in which there are more than 120,000 persons who do not know their right hand from their left, and also much cattle?"* (Jonah 4:10-11). Here, as with Allah, Yahweh has chosen to forgive, but His motive is not inscrutable. Rather, it is clearly identified as the pity He feels for the ignorant and helpless.

Jesus' favorite title for God is "Father," "Heavenly Father", "My Father in Heaven." Christians are encouraged by the Bible to think of God this way, and speak to Him as Father. "Our Father, who art in heaven . . ." (Matthew 6:9). "He (God) chose us in Him before the foundation of the world, that we should be holy and blameless before Him. In love He predestined us for adoption through Jesus Christ" (Ephesians 1:5). He is "the Father, from who every family in heaven and on earth is named" (Ephesians 3:15).

In Islam, to refer to God as one's Father, or even think of Him in such terms, is offensive. It is *shirk*, attempting as a lowly creature to associate oneself with the Ineffable.

So both the nature and character of Yahweh, God as He is revealed in the Bible, and Allah, as he is revealed by Mohammed, are different. In the Bible, love reflects who Yahweh Himself is. In Islam, "love" is the product of the completely free and unpredictable decisions of Allah. Allah chooses whom he will "love."

Jesus. Who is Jesus?

In Islam, Jesus is one of the prophets of Allah who has preceded Mohammed, and whose revelation has therefore been superseded by that given to Mohammed. Jesus' chief message, according to the Koran, was that people should listen to the prophet Ahmed who would come after him. "Ahmed" is a form of the name Mohammed, like "Bill" is a form of "William." The Koran says Jesus should indeed be listened to, for he was, according to the Koran, miraculously born of the Virgin Mary, and lived a sinless life. At the end of history Jesus will return and ask the Christians why they did not believe the message of Mohammed. Jesus did not die on the cross, because Allah would not allow such a thing to happen to his sinless prophet. Rather, Jesus was transported directly to heaven. Jesus is emphatically NOT God. To call a human being God is to commit *shirk*, the worst possible sin. Nor is he the Son of God, because that would mean that God had sex with Mary. So calling Jesus "Son of God," is also *shirk*, horrible sin. It is for believing such things that Muslims believe Christians stand justly condemned. Here are two representative quotes:

> Christians call Christ the son of Allah. That is a saying from their mouth; (in this) they but imitate what the unbelievers of old used to say. Allah's curse be on them: how they are deluded away from the Truth! (Sura 9:30)

> They say:'Allah hath begotten a son!' ... No warrant have ye for this! Say ye about Allah what ye know not? Say: 'Those who invent a lie against Allah will never prosper.' A little enjoyment in this world — and then, to Us will be their return, then shall We make them taste the severest penalty for their blasphemies. (Sura 10:68-70)

The Islamic Jesus is presented in the Qur'an as a preacher of Islamic monotheism who declares hell fire to be the destiny of all who 'associate' anything with Allah:

> They are unbelievers who say:'Allah is the Messiah, Mary's Son.' For the Messiah said: 'Children of Israel, serve Allah, my Lord and your Lord. Verily whoso associates with Allah anything, Allah shall prohibit him entrance to Paradise, and his refuge shall be the Fire; and wrongdoers shall have no helpers.' They are unbelievers who say: Allah is the third of three: for there

is no god except One Allah. If they refrain not from what they say, there shall afflict those of them that disbelieve a painful chastisement. (Sura 5:72-73)

On the other hand, in Christianity, Jesus is God incarnate — God in human form (Colossians 1:15 & 19). Jesus Himself is God's eternal communication of truth to the human race (John 1:1-18). He is "the radiance of the glory of God and the exact imprint of His nature" (Hebrews 1:3).

Actually, there is a parallel in how Christians think of Christ and how Islam presents not Mohammed, but the Koran. Islam teaches that the Koran exists in perfection in heaven. It is called "the Mother of the Book." It is from "the Mother of the Book" that other prophets of the past were given their revelations. But the last, perfect, disclosure from the heavenly Book was given to Mohammed. For Christians, it is not a book called "The Holy Bible" which exists in heaven, but a Person, the Word of God who is the eternal second person of the Trinity, the Holy One who discloses and reveals who God is. By His Holy Spirit this Eternal Word revealed Himself to the prophets of the Old Covenant. But now this same Eternal Word has become a human being, namely Jesus. This same perfect incarnate Word offered Himself on the Cross as the sacrifice in our place, so that both the <u>justice</u> of God which demands punishment for sin, and the <u>love</u> of God, which seeks to save the lost, are fully reconciled in Him, the sinless Man who is also the complete revelation of God in human flesh.

The Source of Spiritual Authority

One source, Mohammed, versus many witnesses

Mohammed is the sole source of authority in Islam. The three texts which are the basis for all Islamic law (sharia), are the Koran, the Hadith, and the Sira. Sometimes you will hear that Islam consists of the Koran and the Sunna. "Sunna" is the term for the life of and traditions about Mohammed. In other words, "Sunna" equals "Hadith" plus "Sira." The Koran is what Mohammed says Allah revealed to him, and only to him. No one else heard the revelations given to Mohammed by Allah. Mohammed never wrote down the revelations he received. All those who believe the Koran must take Mohammed's word for it. The Koran was written later, over time, by those who heard Mohammed. The Hadith are the reported sayings of Mohammed. The Sira is his biography. So everything in Islam is based on what Mohammed did, what Mohammed said, and what Mohammed said Allah said. In the last 10 years of Mohammed's life, as he steadily became the most powerful ruler in Arabia, any questioning of his authority brought his wrath. Submission became the only option.

The Bible, all 66 books of the Old and New Testaments, came into being over at least 1500 years, penned by at least 40 authors, which makes its internal unity all the more remarkable. The Bible texts themselves testify that the teachings of the Bible were resisted and ignored, even by those in the faith community. But then, over and over, unbelief and apostasy become the occasion for deeper revelations of Yahweh's sovereignty, justice, and mercy. For example, the very story of Israel's reluctance to abandon the worship of idols for the pure worship of the one true God becomes a vehicle for Yahweh's further revelation of who He is and what He is like: namely a Savior and a Redeemer. When Jesus comes, he comes as the personification of who Yahweh has already revealed Himself to be precisely because Jesus saves and redeems those who have rejected him. "All we like sheep have gone astray, and turned every one to his own way, and the LORD has laid on him the iniquity of us all" (Isaiah 53:6). This prophecy, which Christians believe to have been fulfilled in Jesus Christ, is completely in keeping with the character of the One God revealed throughout the Bible.

So in Romans 9:25-26 the Apostle Paul quotes the prophet Hosea: *"Those who were not my people I will call 'my people,' and her who was not beloved I will call 'beloved.'"* [26] *"And in the very place where it was said to them, 'You are not my people,' there they will be called 'sons of the living God.'"* (from Hosea 2:23 & 1:10).

Then in Romans 10:20 Paul quotes Isaiah to the same effect: *"I have been found by those who did not seek me; I have shown myself to those who did not ask for me."* (from Isaiah 65:1).

HELPING CHRISTIANS UNDERSTAND *Islam*

Jesus affirms this same aspect of Yahweh's character: "*Love your enemies, and do good . . . and you will be sons of the Most High, for he is kind to the ungrateful and the evil*" (Luke 6:35).

In the case of Mohammed, Mohammed's lone voice testifies to Allah, who is ultimately unknowable, and who "loves" only those who submit to him. In the case of the Bible, many voices testify to Yahweh, the "I Am," who from the beginning loves His human children and wants them to know Him.

Reliability of the texts we have

It is a standard claim of Islam that the Jewish and Christian scriptures are corrupted. Only what Allah has revealed to Mohammed is reliable. But when we compare the history of transmission of the text of the Bible with both the Koran and Hadith, it seems the case is rather the reverse.

The majority of Old Testament manuscripts we have preserve the "Masoretic Text," the text of the Jewish Masoretic scholars, who devised elaborate systems for checking that they were copying the Word of God without mistakes. Thanks to the Dead Sea Scrolls, we now have Old Testament manuscripts many centuries older than the "Masoretic Text," and these older manuscripts demonstrate that the text of the Old Testament was altered very little over centuries of copying. Careful scholarship confirms the reliability of the Old Testament text we have today.

The New Testament is even more strongly established. We have more manuscripts for the New Testament than for any other ancient document. The discrepancies are few and well known, such as the ending of the Gospel of Mark. None affect the doctrines of the Christian faith. Much scholarship has been expended to give us a Greek text of the New Testament that is virtually the same as that produced by the original authors. Those authors either were themselves Apostles, the witnesses to the Resurrection, or they wrote during the lifetime of those Apostles. The churches in their day received what the New Testament authors wrote as true.

Muslim critics who claim the Christian scriptures are corrupted have a bit of a dilemma to solve. If the corruption occurred since the time of Mohammed, then why do the Old and New Testament manuscripts that predate Mohammed agree with the later ones? But if the corruption occurred before the time of Mohammed, then why does the Koran commend the scriptures of the Christians? As, for instance, in **Surat Al-M'idah (The Table Spread) -5:68** Yusuf Ali Translation: **"Say: 'O People of the Book! ye have no ground to stand upon unless ye stand fast by the Law, the Gospel, and all the revelation that has come to you from your Lord.' It is the revelation that cometh to thee from thy Lord, that increaseth in most of them their obstinate rebellion and blasphemy. But sorrow thou not over (these) people (who are) without Faith."** In the above verse Christians are commanded in the Qur'an to continue holding on to the Scriptures if they want to stand on the day of the judgment. This verse alone invalidates the Islamic claim that the Christian scriptures are corrupt.

In the case of the Koran, there are fewer ancient manuscripts than we have for the Bible because Uthman, the Third Caliph (supreme Muslim ruler), destroyed most of the ones that existed at the time of his caliphate (644-656), and decreed that the manuscripts he had preserved were the correct ones, agreeing exactly with what was dictated to Mohammed by Allah through the angel Gabriel. However, there have long been some disagreements over the Koran text. The minority Shi'a Muslims accept two chapters (Sura) as original which the majority Sunni Muslims do not. Further, beginning in 1972, ancient copies of the Koran were found in a mosque in Yemen. These Korans contain significant textual differences from the "standard" Koran.

This poses a problem for Muslim theology. The Koran as Mohammed received it is dictated perfectly from heaven in Arabic. Even translating it makes it no longer the Koran. What then to do with varying manuscripts?

The Christian understanding of inspiration does not face the same difficulties. Rather than God dictating word-for-word what the Bible's writers should say, Christians understand that the Holy Spirit guided the writers so that the content of what they wrote was what God intended. Because the content of a message can be translated, translations of the Bible are also, for Christians, the Word of God.

On the issue of the Hadith, the "sayings" of Mohammed, they were collected and put into writing more than 200 years after Mohammed's death. The Sira, Mohammed's biography, was written more than 100 years after his death. Keep in mind that the Hadith and Sira, because they give the sayings and behavior of Mohammed, are authoritative sources for Muslim law, *sharia*. Many practices of Islam are not found in the Koran, but only in the Hadith or Sira.

Moral content, abrogation, and purpose

As mentioned in the first chapter, the Koran, particularly those parts from Mohammed's time in Medina, makes a sharp distinction between Muslims and *kafirs*, the insulting word which refers to all those who do not accept Mohammed as Allah's prophet. In other words, there are two different systems of ethics: one for fellow-Muslims and another for *kafirs*. Some other distinctions in the moral content of the Bible and the Koran include:

✦ **the treatment of women**

✦ **the relationship of religious faith to politics**

✦ **other required behaviors**

In upcoming chapters, we'll examine these in more detail, but even what has been said already shows clearly that what Allah revealed to Mohammed and what the Biblical authors believed and taught are quite different.

One tricky issue that we should deal with here is the Muslim doctrine of **abrogation**. This, remember, is the doctrine that where Allah in the Koran declares two contradictory things, such as on the one hand tolerating Jews and Christians (*Sura 73:10*) and on the other hand cutting off their heads and the tips of their fingers (*Sura 8:12*), the later verse *abrogates* or cancels out the first. Later words of Allah take precedence over words he spoke earlier. For example, all the "friendly" verses about Jews and Christians which are part of the Meccan Koran are abrogated by the verses of the Medinan Koran which express hatred toward them. But since all the words of the Koran, even the abrogated ones, are the words of God, all of them can be used in the cause of advancing Islam. So when it is helpful to quote the friendly words about Jews and Christians, it is quite proper to do so.

At first glance, it would seem that Christianity does the same thing. After all, the New Testament replaces the Old Testament. Or does it? When Jesus says, speaking of commandments of the Old Testament: "You have heard it said to those of old . . . but I say to you" (Matthew 5:21 and following), he is taking a commandment and expanding its scope to include wrong thoughts and attitudes, not just external actions. He explicitly begins this section in Matthew by saying: "Do not think I have come to abolish the Law or the Prophets; I have not come to abolish them but to fulfill them" (Matthew 5:17). As a different example, the animal sacrifices which God required of Israel are no longer needed because Christ came and offered Himself as the perfect eternal sacrifice. But the verses in the Old Testament where God commands the sacrifices are not abrogated, or negated. Rather they continue to serve their original function, which was to anticipate or foreshadow what God would do in Christ. So the Old Testament is not abrogated for Christians. But, someone may say, what about those places in the Old Testament where God changes His mind? Well, let's take a famous one. God tells Jonah to go preach to Nineveh and tell them their city is going to be destroyed. Then God overrules Himself and doesn't do it. Is that the same as abrogation? No, because Jonah knows all along that God's reason for having Jonah preach destruction is so that destruction will not come, but rather that Nineveh will repent and be saved. God's intention is consistent throughout the story, and consistent with His character throughout the Bible. Because He loves people, His aim is always to save them if they are willing. So nothing in the Bible is "abrogated" in the sense in which the term is used in the Koran.

Abrogation in the Koran works differently. The earlier and later verses which contradict each other ("tolerate Jews and Christians" vs. "behead Jews and Christians"), are BOTH the Word of God. Both are to be done. The issue is: which verse will do the most to advance Islam at a particular time, that is, bring people into submission to Allah and his prophet? The same can even be said of the famous "Satanic Verses," the subject of Salman Rushdie's novel of that name, where Allah tells Mohammed it is ok for the Meccans to have their idols intercede with Allah for them, but then later Allah tells Mohammed that these verses were inspired by Satan. The "Satanic Verses" are there in the Koran to be used to advance Islam. But for them to be used to denigrate Islam, as Salman Rushdie did in his book about them, calls for the harshest punishment.

Any use of the Koran, or the Hadith, or the example of Mohammed's life, that produces criticism of Allah, of Islam, or of Allah's prophet, is illegitimate. Any use which exalts Allah, Islam, or Allah's prophet is commendable, according to the sacred texts themselves. The purpose for which Mohammed was called by Allah, and the purpose for which the Koran was given, is to produce Islam, submission to Allah as his will is revealed by his prophet Mohammed.

In contrast, the purpose of the Bible is to invite human beings to turn from sin and put their trust in Jesus Christ to save them, entering into the relationship with God that He intended from the beginning.

Human Nature

Another area where Islam and Christianity do not agree is their understanding of human nature. In the Christian understanding, God created man and woman in His image, with the intention that they, in direct communication with Him, be His vice-regents over the rest of His creation (Gen. 1:26-28). But through disobedience, sin entered into the world, and with it, death (Romans 5:12). The entire human race is under bondage to sin and death (Romans 5:14). The heart, the center of human personality, is diseased with sin. "The heart is deceitful above all things, and desperately wicked. Who can know it?" (Jeremiah 17:9)

But in Islam, to say humans are "created in Allah's image" is *shirk*, terrible sin, because it is impossible that anything in Creation conveys his image. One cannot even say that anything in Creation is "like" him. So human beings do not have the dignity of being God's image-bearers in Islam.

On the other hand, in Islam the human race is not fallen. Individuals do commit sin, yes, but human nature has not been corrupted by the Fall. In Islam, Adam's sin caused his expulsion from the garden, but each subsequent human starts with a "blank slate" as far as sin is concerned. Human beings are capable of obedience to Allah, therefore they must submit to him without excuse.

A way to sum up the difference between Christianity and Islam on the question of human nature is to say that Christianity teaches that people are born naturally "bent" toward sin. Islam teaches that people are born with an unblemished nature that is equally capable of sin or good deeds. But as the French Christian philosopher Blaise Pascal pointed out, while the concept of original sin is difficult to understand, it is even more difficult to make sense of the corrupt history of the human race without it. If the human "default mode" is not sin, why is it universally prevalent?

The Way of Salvation

It is the desperate condition of the human race, "dead in trespasses and sins" (Ephesians 2:1), that makes it impossible for us to rescue ourselves. We need help, help from Someone who is not in bondage to sin. We need a Savior.

> "For I am the LORD your God, the Holy One of Israel, your **Savior**" (**Isaiah 43:3**).

> "you **shall** call **his** name **Jesus** (**Jeshua, the LORD** saves), for he will **save his people** from their sins" (**Matthew 1:21**).

> "All have sinned and fall short of the glory of God" (**Romans 3:23**).

So what is the solution provided by the God of the Bible? Those who have sinned "are justified by his grace as a gift, through the redemption that is in Christ Jesus, whom God put forward as a propitiation (a sacrificial payment) by his blood, to be received by faith. This was to show God's righteousness, because in his divine forbearance he had passed over former sins. It was to

HELPING CHRISTIANS UNDERSTAND *Islam*

show his righteousness at the present time, so that he might be just and the justifier of the one who has faith in Jesus." (**Romans 3:24-26**).

Jesus took our place and received the punishment due us. God's justice is satisfied, because our sin is paid for. All we need do is accept what Jesus has done for us when He gave Himself up for us. This is what it means to be saved by faith. I am not trusting in what I have done to save myself. Nor do I condemn myself because of my sins. Instead, I trust in what Jesus has done for me to save me. "In my hand no price I bring, **simply to Thy cross I cling**" (Toplady, *Rock of Ages*).

In Islam, while it is certainly necessary to believe that Allah is exactly as Mohammed has declared him, what saves is not what Mohammed nor anyone else has done for you. It is whether you have been obedient to Allah. Obedience includes the "5 Pillars," namely, 1) saying the *Shahada*, "There is no God but Allah, and Mohammed is the prophet of Allah," 2) praying 5 times daily, 3) fasting during the month of Ramadan, 4) giving charity (to Muslims and Muslim causes only), and 5) making the pilgrimage to Mecca. In addition, *jihad*, striving to advance the cause of Allah by whatever means are open to one, is also commanded of all Muslims. Then in addition, there are numerous detailed ordinances which cover every aspect of personal life, family life, society, and politics. Many of these are laid out in the handbook on *sharia*, Islamic law, entitled <u>The Reliance of the Traveler</u>.[1] This has been helpfully translated into English for anyone who would like to know in detail what Islam requires.

The difficulty with all this is that no matter how faithful a Muslim one has been, one has no assurance of entering Paradise after death. One's bad deeds may well outweigh one's good deeds, causing one to fall into the lake of fire. Ultimately, one's eternal fate is entirely at the sole discretion of Allah. Mohammed taught that he did not know if he himself would enter Paradise. The best hope for entering Paradise, however, is to perish in the cause of Allah. That is, to die while practicing *jihad*.

Here is an example from the Hadith:

> Narrated Abu Huraira:
> The Prophet said, "The person who participates in (Holy battles) in Allah's cause and nothing compels him to do so

except belief in Allah and His Apostles, will be recompensed by Allah either with a reward, or booty (if he survives) or will be admitted to Paradise (if he is killed in the battle as a martyr). Had I not found it difficult for my followers, then I would not remain behind any *sariya* going for Jihad and I would have loved to be martyred in Allah's cause and then made alive, and then martyred and then made alive, and then again martyred in His cause." (*Sahih al-Bukhari 1.35*, also *Sahih al-Bukhari 4.386*)

So in Islam, salvation, if it is to be found at all, is found by doing what Allah commands, and doing battle for Allah brings the highest reward from him. This brings us to the inescapably dominant role of what Bill Warner calls "Political Islam." (www.politicalislam.com). Using this term helps us understand that the bulk of Islamic teaching is not "religion" in the sense that we understand the term, but political ideology and practice. However, we must keep in mind that the areas correctly described as "political" are just as much a part of Islam as the areas we would call "religious." That is, how one treats *kafirs* is just as important in Islam, if not more so, than praying correctly five times a day.

Political Islam is the majority of the teachings found in the Medinan Koran, the Hadith, and the Sira. A major block of texts: 24% of the entire Koran from the Medina period, 21% of all the Hadith, and 67% of the Sira, Mohammed's life, deal with jihad against non-Muslims, for whom there is the special denigrating term: *kafir*. All struggle to bring kafirs into submission to Islam is jihad. In the light of this, we will examine:

✦ Jews and Christians in Islam

✦ Dhimmis and Slaves

✦ Ethics and Women

✦ Triumphs and Tears

Prior to the 9/11 attacks, Osama Bin Laden wrote a letter to America, where he explained that "it is to this religion (Islam) that we call you; the seal of all the previous religions....It is the religion of showing kindness to others, establishing justice between them, granting them their rights, and defending the oppressed and the persecuted....It is the religion of Jihad in the way of Allah so that Allah's Word and religion reign Supreme." In subsequent chapters we'll learn better what Bin Laden meant by this.

QUESTIONS:

1. Many Americans believe that "all religions teach the same thing." What are three points from this chapter that highlight the different teachings of Christianity and Islam?

2. Which scripture appears to you to be more reliable, the Koran or the Bible? Why?

3. Mohammed was much more successful after he went to Medina. What contributed to this?

Endnotes:

1   Revised edition, Edited & Translated by Nuh Ha Mim Keller, Amana Publications, Beltsville, MD 1991, 1994.

Chapter 3
Jews and Christians in Political Islam

In the next four chapters of this book, the focus will be on what Bill Warner calls "Political Islam." (www.politicalislam.com) Using this term helps us understand that the bulk of Islamic teaching is not "religion" in the sense that we understand the term, but political ideology and practice. This is in marked contrast to the Bible. There are many Biblical doctrines, such as the *imago Dei* (image of God) and the Golden Rule, which have deeply impacted the laws and mores of countries which have had Christianity as their majority religion. But the Bible's focus is not to lay out a political program.

This has allowed Christianity to be practiced under many different political systems. Sometimes it has been in tension with them, as in the early Roman Empire, or under Soviet Communism. At other times it has fit more or less well with the existing political system, as in the "Christendom" of medieval Europe, or the American democratic republic of the 19th century. But in no case has any political system been identified as "the" Christian political system, because, unlike Islam, Christianity does not include a specific political ideology.

What is the difference between religious Islam and political Islam? Remember that when some Danish artists drew some cartoons of Mohammed there were weeks of rioting, threats, lawsuits, killings, assassinations and destruction by Muslims. If Muslims want to respect Mohammed by never criticizing, never joking about him and by taking every word he said as a sacred example, that is religious. But when they threaten, pressure and hurt non-Muslims for not respecting Mohammed, that is political. When Muslims say that Mohammed is the prophet of the only god, that is religious, but when they insist that non-Muslims never disrespect Mohamed, that is political. When the newspapers and TV agreed not to publish the cartoons, that decision was a political response, not a religious response. The publishers and station owners were not following their religious convictions, they were bowing to political pressure, including threats of violence.

We can contrast this with the Christian response when a so-called artist displayed a crucified Christ in a vat of urine in a public museum in Brooklyn, NY, at public expense. Christians wrote letters to the editor and held up signs outside the museum, but did not engage in any violence. That was the extent of their political response to the offensive "artist." The reason for this is grounded in Christianity's authoritative text, the Bible. Jesus famously said: "My kingdom is not of this world" (John 18:36). In fact, the Gospels depict world political leadership as a temptation from Satan that Jesus explicitly rejects (Matthew 4:8-10; Luke 4:5-8). Moreover, Jesus taught His followers: "Blessed are you when others revile you and persecute you and utter all kinds of evil against you falsely on my account. Rejoice and be glad, for your reward is great in heaven." (Matt. 5:11). He also taught them: "if anyone slaps you on the right cheek, turn to him the other also . . . Love your enemies and pray for those who persecute you" (Matt. 5:39, 44).

Political Islam makes up the majority of the teachings found in the Medina Koran, the Hadith, and the Sira. A great many of the texts: 24% of the entire Koran from the Medina period, 21% of all the Hadith, and 67% of the Sira, Mohammed's life, deal with jihad against non-Muslims.[1] Mohammed introduced a special denigrating term for non-Muslims: *kafir*.

All struggle to bring kafirs into submission to Islam is jihad. In the light of this, we will first examine Jews and Christians in Islam.

The Jews[2]

The Jews are very important in the formation of Islam. It could be said that if there were no Jews there would be no Islam. The reason for this can be found in the Koran. When Mohammed had his first vision, which no one else saw, and when he heard the voices that no one else heard, he said that the voice was that of the Angel Gabriel. This is important because Gabriel is in the Jewish tradition. From the beginning Mohammed said that his authenticity had the same basis as the prophets in the Old Testament. When he started telling his versions of the stories of Noah and Adam and Moses to people in Mecca, there were no Jews there who had heard the original version, which was already some 2000+ years old in Mohammed's day. In the Koran's version, the characters are the same but the stories are different. For instance in the Jewish scriptures, the story of Moses and the Pharaoh is about the release of the Jewish slaves. In the Koran, the story of Moses and the Pharaoh is not about freeing the Jews; instead the story says that the Egyptians were destroyed because Pharaoh would not admit that Moses was a prophet of Allah.

In the story of Noah, the same pattern continues. The reason that Allah destroyed the Earth with water was because men would not believe that Noah was a prophet of Allah. The words with which Noah's opponents attack him, according to the Koran, are expressions like this: **"He is only a madman; be patient with him for a while."** Interestingly, in the Koran the *kafirs* of Noah's day use the same expressions attacking Noah that the Meccans do in attacking Mohammed. In every case the Biblical story is changed so as to advance the Koran's central argument that everyone must listen and do exactly what a prophet of Allah says. In the Koran the entire world is divided into those who believe and obey Mohammed, the prophet Allah has sent, and those who do not.

So in the Koran, the Jews are portrayed favorably at first. But listen to what modern Muslim political leaders have to say today about the Jews in the modern world. A former Turkish Prime Minister in front of crowds publicly proclaimed that "the Jews are bacteria and like a disease". In Saudi Arabia on a TV show an interviewer asked "the man on the street" questions about the Jews. One of them was: "Would you be willing to shake hands with a Jew?" One person said "Of course not. I would have to cut off my hand." Another question: "If a child asked you who were the Jews what would you say?" One respondent: "Allah's anger is upon them. They strayed from the path of righteousness; they are the filthiest people on the face of the earth because they only care about themselves."

Another quote is from a modern Muslim who is a professor in a university in Egypt that is the Islamic equivalent to Harvard. This imam is on a fatwa committee; that is, a committee that makes legal judgments binding on Muslims. This professor reported that the committee issued a fatwa saying that Jews were "apes and pigs." They went further to say that Jews "fabricate lies, they listen to lies, and they hide the truth and support deception. They are hypocrites. They want other people to feel pain. They are happy when others suffer. They are rude and vulgar. They break their promises and they're cowards."

This is a decided contrast to Mohammed in Mecca. In Mecca Mohammed told the reworked stories of the Jewish prophets to prove that he was a real prophet like them. He said that he was the last of the line of the Jewish prophets. What explains this sharp discrepancy? Some people think that Muslims picked up their hatred of Jews from Europeans, that it's a remnant of the Christianity of the Middle Ages, or of Nazism. Let's examine this further by going back to the Koran and the example of Mohammed.

As mentioned in Chapter I, there are, for all practical purposes, two Korans. The second Koran, the part written in Medina during the last 10 years of Mohammed's life, draws a totally different picture of the Jews than the earlier part written in Mecca. When Mohammed reached Medina after leaving Mecca, he found a lot of Jews in Medina. There were three Jewish tribes when Mohammed arrived there in 622 AD, and they comprised about half the population. So when Mohammed entered Medina and began preaching it did not take long for the Jews to inform him that he was not a prophet in the line of the Hebrew prophets. Mohammed soon proved that they were correct, because the Old Testament is full of stories of true prophets of Yahweh suffering unjustly. In neither Old nor New Testament does a messenger of God initiate revenge for wrongs committed against himself. But Allah's prophet Mohammed was different. No one was allowed to contradict Mohammed, so after about a year in Medina, when he had become politically powerful enough, he attacked one of the Jewish tribes. He defeated them and took all of their money and exiled them from Medina. Not long after that, he found an excuse to attack the second Jewish tribe. After he captured them he took all of their wealth and was going to do worse. But these Jews had allies among the Arabs. One of their old allies stepped forth and said "do not harm them; they are former allies of mine." So Mohammed exiled them and took all of their money.

His third attack was against the strongest tribe of Jews. After the Jews surrendered, the men were separated from the women and children. The men were taken into the marketplace and one by one their heads were cut off, all 800 of them. Mohammed sat there throughout the day sitting beside his 12-year-old wife Aisha. The executions went on into the night. By 10 o'clock at night the last Jew lost his head by torchlight. The Jewish women and children were taken into Muslim families and raised as Muslims or else sold into slavery. This is a story clearly recounted in Mohammed's biography, the Sira, which makes up a part of the foundation of Islamic law. After the Jews of Medina had been destroyed, Mohammed did not stop there.

He went north to Khaybar where the Jews were prosperous. He put them under siege, and after they surrendered he took all of their wealth. But this time he did not kill them, because he wanted their income. Instead, Mohammed created a new form of human being called the *dhimmi*. A *dhimmi* is an alien in an Islamic world. A Jew who was a *dhimmi* could henceforth only be Jewish in his home or in the synagogue. All of the surrounding culture was Islamic, including the laws and the political system. The *dhimmis* had to pay a tax, the *jizya*. 50% of everything they earned was paid to Islam and Mohammed. The Koran decreed that in addition to paying the tax *dhimmis* must be humiliated.

But Mohammed did not stop with making *dhimmis* of the Jews of Khaybar. As he lay on his deathbed, his last words were that neither Jew nor Christian should be allowed in Arabia. Three years after that, when Umar was caliph, supreme ruler of all of Islam, he drove the Jews out of Arabia. From that day forward there have been no Jews in Arabia. Saudi Arabia exists in religious apartheid.

The Koran goes further in talking about the Jews; it calls them "apes." Remember the modern fatwa that ruled that the Jews are apes and pigs? The modern imams didn't invent those terms. Mohammed added further that the Jews were rats. So within the Koran are two totally different views of the Jews. This is a dramatic example of the duality one finds throughout Islam. One view of the Jews is that Jews and Muslims worship the same God. Why, they are both children of Abraham! The other view of the Jews is they are "apes and rats." A Muslim can say to the Jew, "Oh, we worship the same God. We are brothers in religion." Or he can say that Jews are apes and rats. These are two opposite ideas, but due to the duality within Islam they are both considered correct.

We've briefly reviewed the history of Jews under Islam and seen that Mohammed enslaved and killed Jews and created the concept of "*dhimmi*." In that one word, *dhimmi*, we find the reason that Jews and Christians do not recognize the source of their problems in Islam. Wherever Islam has come into power they have been annihilated, humiliated and shamed. Wherever Islam came, Jews and Christians were *dhimmis*. Whether it was Persia, North Africa, Spain, Turkey or Egypt; *dhimmis* were treated badly. No one chooses to remember such dreadful history; it's simpler to ignore it.

In fact, one can well argue that what is often called "anti-Semitism," or, more accurately, "Jew hatred," began with Mohammed. He is the first person to elevate hatred of Jews to the status of a doctrine given by divine revelation. For example, in the biblical book of Esther, Haman certainly hated the Jews, but did so because of his personal envy. But according to Mohammed, Allah declares that Jews are apes, pigs, and rats. It is Allah who commands Muslims to destroy them before the Last Day. It is Allah who commanded that Jews be the first persons reduced to *dhimmi* status, a status which was then extended to all *kafirs*.

Instead of telling this 1400-year history of shame, modern scholars, including Jewish scholars, create a beautiful story, the story of a golden age of Islam. It is even said that the high point of civilization was found in Islamic Spain, and that it was a culture of tolerance with great intellectual ferment. There is some truth to this, in that there were some Jews and Christians who prospered and were in high places of government as advisers and in other capacities. But to call this a golden age is an elitist view, because only a Jewish and Christian elite prospered. Can a golden age exist that is based upon the slavery or dhimmitude of multiple thousands of kafirs? Can it be a golden age when the Europeans strove for seven hundred years to drive out Islam from Spain? Can a Jewish scholar speak of a golden age when 5000 Jews could be killed in one day in Cordoba? Or 4000 in one day in Granada? The sins of medieval Christendom against Jews are well known. The treatment of Jews by medieval Islam deserves to be better known, not covered over or sugar-coated.

It is the history of the *dhimmi* that explains our historical amnesia about the history of Islam and the Jews. No kafir: Jewish, Christian, Hindu, Buddhist, or animist, wants to look back and see how a total of some 270 million kafirs have been killed over 1400 years in the name of Islam. The history is too dreadful. No kafir wants to look back and say that his ancestors were enslaved. No Jew wants to look back and say that for 1400 years Jews were regarded as dirt on the street in Islam. Many stories about how Jews were treated exist in Muslim sources. Here are some examples:

✦ In Tunisia when the call to prayer came a Jew said that Mohammed was no prophet in the line of the Jews. He was beheaded for insulting the prophet. A Jew who dressed like a Muslim was to be stripped and beaten and jailed. If he was caught riding a horse he was to be pulled off of the horse, stripped, and beaten.

✦ In North Africa Jews that sold wine to Muslims were beheaded and their families sold into slavery.

✦ In medieval Iran, a Jew was forbidden to go out into the rain since the water might fall off him onto the ground and a Muslim might step in it and become contaminated. So as a consequence when it rained, Jews were not allowed in the marketplace for fear of contaminating Muslims.

It is sad that this history is not remembered, and that the modern relations between Israel and its Islamic neighbors is never viewed through the lens of this history, but only through what has happened since 1948.[3]

Modern historians know about, and recount, the bad treatment Jews received in Medieval Europe, such as their wholesale expulsion from some countries, including France and Spain. It is right that this shameful history should be known. But let's also ask the question: why does such self-criticism arise in countries whose cultural heritage is Christian, but never in Islamic countries or societies? The perspective to look at Medieval Europe and criticize its treatment of the Jews arose in Christianity, not in Islam. But before we consider why this is true, what about Christians? How does Islam see them?

The Christians[4]

Islam has two views of Christians (duality again). The first view is that Christianity and Islam are brother religions. The second view is that Christians must change their religion to meet the demands of Islam. Modern Christians want to believe that there is a bridge between Islam and Christianity. For example, in 2007 138 Muslim scholars wrote an open letter to Christians, and four Yale scholars wrote a welcoming response and got 300 Christian leaders to sign it. Unfortunately, the Yale scholars were apparently unaware of the history of such seemingly-friendly letters from Muslim leaders.[5] Such letters in the past have been part of a history of Islam where Islam first deceives and then annihilates Christianity. There is even an Islamic term for invitations to Islam: *da'wa*. The original version of such a letter was written by Muhammad himself as a declaration of war to the Eastern Roman (Byzantine) Emperor, Heraclius. Bukhari's collection of hadith, the most prestigious in Sunni Islam, gives the text of this letter in the *Book of Jihad*, hadith No. 2940:

> In the name of Allah, the most Gracious, the most Merciful. (This letter is) from Muhammad, the slave of Allah, and His Messenger, to Heraclius, the Ruler of the Byzantines. Peace be upon him, who follows the (true) guidance. Now then, I invite you to Islam (i.e. surrender to Allah), embrace Islam and you will be safe [*aslim taslam*]; embrace Islam and Allah will bestow on you a double reward. But if you reject this invitation of Islam, you shall be responsible for misguiding the peasants (i.e. your nation). *O people of the Scriptures (Jews and Christians)! Come to a word that is just between us and you, that we worship none but Allah, and that we associate no partners with him; and that none of us shall take lords besides Allah. Then if they turn away, say: Bear witness that we are Muslims.* (3.64)

This hadith is included in the *Book of Jihad* because it illustrates Mohammad's principle that, before attacking non-Muslims, it was necessary first to invite them to embrace Islam. The message *aslim taslam* "surrender (or 'embrace Islam') and you will be safe" is an essential component of a declaration of war in Islam. Osam Bin Laden was following the example of Mohammed in the letter he wrote to America before the 9/11 attacks, the letter quoted at the end of Chapter 2. The seemingly-friendly open letter to Christians to which the Yale scholars responded in genuine good will is another example of such a letter.

For 1400 years Islam has invited Christians to enter Islam, and, when they have not, has attacked them and taken over their lands.

Christians did not play a pivotal role like the Jews did in the formation of Islam. That is, the Koran does not have as much to say about Christians, although the early part of the Koran, the part Mohammed declared in Mecca, calls them "People of the Book," like the Jews. Nor does the Sira, the life of Mohammed, have much to say about Christians, although it describes Christians arguing the doctrine of the Trinity with Mohammed. The Koran does explicitly deny the divinity of Jesus, and says that the Christian Trinity is Allah, Jesus, and Mary. But Mohammed's attitude toward Christians, and therefore Islam's official attitude, can be seen in some of the final days of Mohammed's life when he sent out troops against the Christians in the North of Syria, showing it was his intent to attack the Christians. Soon after he died that's what happened, beginning under Umar, the second Caliph. Since then, Christians have played a very important role in the history of Islam and the reason is that all the Middle East including Persia (Iran), North Africa, and what we now call Turkey was formerly Christian until the rise of Islam.

Since these areas are Islamic today, there is a history there, and it did not start with the Crusades. Yes, mistakes were made in the Crusades, and much was done that was morally wrong, as in every war ever fought. But the Crusades were one of the few times the Christians in Europe recognized the intense suffering of the Christians in the Middle East. The reasons the Crusades were started were simple. They came as a response to a cry for help. And why did these Christians cry for help? Because they were being murdered, robbed and taxed to death by their Muslim overlords.

How did these Muslims become their overlords? Originally that part of the world had been mostly Christian. It did not become Islamic because some imams showed up and started preaching in the marketplace. No, it was Islamic because the sword had been used to kill all those who would defend Christianity and to take over the government, and the surviving population was oppressed as *dhimmis*. The Crusaders arrived in response to a desperate cry for help.

Over 60 million Christians have been killed in the process of jihad. How did Turkey, for example, which is 99.7 percent Islamic, go from an Orthodox Christian culture to an Islamic culture? In the 20th century alone 1.5 million Armenians who belonged to the Orthodox Church were killed in Turkey.

Why don't they teach this at the universities and divinity schools? The reason that Christians don't teach the history of Christianity and Islam is this: it is so dreadful, so painful, even disgusting, so much so that it is difficult to believe it actually happened. The process whereby the Middle East and Turkey and North Africa all became Muslim was so tragic. There's nothing positive or encouraging about it. It is a history of unmitigated suffering and defeat.

Islam's political status for Christians under Muslim control is that of *dhimmis*. The Jews, remember, were the first *dhimmis*, but the Christians became the biggest number of *dhimmis* for the simple reason that there were far more of them. When the Muslims came in and took over the government of Christian-majority areas and implemented Islamic *sharia* law, part of this dictated how Christians and Jews would be treated in public and how they would be treated in the courts of law. It was dreadful. A *dhimmi* has no civil rights. The whole idea of "civil rights" arose in cultures influenced by Christianity. So a history of *dhimmitude*, including public humiliation and special taxes, was deeply humiliating. It wasn't something Christian writers who were contemporaries of these events were proud of repeating, just as modern Christian writers mostly shy away from describing the persecution of Christians today in Muslim-majority areas.[6]

In the book of Revelation in the New Testament, the seven churches of Asia are addressed. The seven churches were in Asia Minor, what we call Turkey today. That Christians don't know what happened to those churches is a real tragedy. Those Christians became part of the 60 million Christians murdered during the expansion of Islam. The destruction of those churches is the history of Islamic expansion in miniature.

And Christians do not know enough about Islam to know that not only have over 60 million Christians been killed in jihad, but also 80 million Hindus, 10 million Buddhists and 120 million Africans.

All Christians should know enough about the Koran that when a Muslim says Christians, Jews and Muslims worship the same God, they can explain why this cannot be true. Yes, Christians, Jews, and Muslims are all monotheists. They believe in one Supreme Being. But the nature and character of the God revealed in the Bible and the nature and character of Allah as revealed by Mohammed are very, very different. This knowledge is available for those with the courage to embrace it. Yahweh, the LORD God of the Bible, commands the preaching of the truth to those who do not believe in Him. But all are free not to believe. Judgment for unbelief is an eternal, not a temporal, matter. But Allah, whose prophet is Mohammed, commands that all must submit to Mohammed's revelation, or else be killed, enslaved, or become *dhimmis*. Judgment for unbelief is to take place in this life as well as the next.

All kafirs, including Christians, need to be able to explain political Islam, not just in speaking with a Muslim, but when the subject comes up at work or wherever else. Each of us must face the uneasy feeling, or even fear, that we may feel when dealing factually with political Islam, because the dreadful history of Islam is repeating itself in our world today. As an example, Iraq, which used to be a majority Christian country, is now only 3% Christian, and yet of the refugees leaving Iraq, 30% of those leaving are Christian. Why is it that they're being persecuted? They are certainly not numerous enough to be any threat to a Muslim-majority government. No, a 1400 year old history is repeating itself today in Iraq. And lest someone think this is solely due to American intervention in Iraq, we also have modern Africa. In Africa today, in places where there is no American presence, Christian Africans are being killed and destroyed almost on a daily basis. The article in Appendix I gives a good example of this. Where the Christians are numerous enough, as in Nigeria or Sudan, they fight back, and civil conflict breaks out.

Moreover, what has been done to Christians has been done to Jews, Hindus, Buddhists and atheists. Islam does not discriminate. Here, for example is a quote from the *Sacramento Bee* newspaper, May 15, 2011: *"More than 4,200 people have been killed in predominantly Buddhist Thailand's three Muslim-dominated southern provinces since an Islamist insurgency erupted here in 2004."* http://www.sacbee.com/2011/05/16/3629168/thai-bomb-attack-in-south-kills.html#ixzz1MYDsvHyQ

There is no American military occupation of southern Thailand. But there are Muslims acting according to the example of Mohammed, eliminating kafirs, who happen to be Buddhist in this case. The bottom line is the same; all kafirs must submit.

Now, someone may well say: "Christians have done terrible things, too, especially to Jews." And unfortunately, that is correct. Here is something constant in persecutions of the Jews or any other minority; when any group has exclusive political ascendancy, it seldom resists the temptation to treat minority groups badly. This is true whether the group in power is an ethnic or a religious one. So Christians with dominant political power, as in Medieval Christendom in Europe, have acted badly toward minorities. What is encouraging, though, is that it is possible to find significant exceptions, places where Christians controlled the political situation, but exercised tolerance toward religious minorities, not just toward favored elite individuals within minority religions. A famous example is George Washington's letter to the Jewish synagogue in Newport, RI. Here's what he wrote them:

> "May the children of the stock of Abraham who dwell in this land continue to merit and enjoy the good will of the other inhabitants while every one shall sit in safety under his own vine and fig tree and there shall be none to make him afraid.
>
> May the father of all mercies scatter light, and not darkness, upon our paths, and make us all in our several vocations useful here, and in His own due time and way everlastingly happy."
>
> G. *Washington*

Washington's letter contains a clue as to where Christian-dominated governments can and have found the basis of tolerance for other religions, and shows why America, with a large nominally-Christian majority, has been a political haven for Jews. Washington quotes and paraphrases the Bible. That is, in the founding document of Christianity one does not find a basis for persecuting those of another religion simply because of what they believe, nor any basis for relegating them to second-class political status. This runs very deeply throughout the Bible narrative.

> [26]*Then God said, "Let us make man in our image, after our likeness. And let them have dominion over the fish of the sea and over the birds of the heavens and over the livestock and over all the earth and over every creeping thing that creeps on the earth."*

²⁷*So God created man in his own image, in the image of God he created him; male and female he created them. Gen. 1:26-27*

All human beings are made in God's image, hence all are of equal inherent worth. This same principle is upheld in the law of the people of Israel.

Leviticus 24:22 (speaking of equal enforcement of the law)

*"You shall have the same rule for the **sojourner** and for the native, for I am the LORD your God."*

Numbers 9:14 (non-Jews are invited to the most sacred festival)

*"And if a stranger sojourns among you and would keep the Passover to the LORD, according to the statute of the Passover and according to its rule, so shall he do. You shall have one statute, both for the **sojourner** and for the native."*

Numbers 15:15 (non-Jews are invited to participate in worship)

*"For the assembly, there shall be one statute for you and for the stranger who sojourns with you, a statute forever throughout your generations. You and the **sojourner** shall be alike before the LORD."*

Moreover, Yahweh, the LORD, intends to reconcile the nations so as to bring peace:

Isaiah 2:2-4

²*It shall come to pass in the latter days that the mountain of the house of the LORD shall be established as the highest of the mountains, and shall be lifted up above the hills; and all the nations shall flow to it,*

³*and many peoples shall come, and say: "Come, let us go up to the mountain of the LORD, to the house of the God of Jacob, that he may teach us his ways and that we may walk in his paths." For out of Zion shall go the law, and the word of the LORD from Jerusalem.*

⁴*He shall judge between the nations, and shall decide disputes for many peoples; and they shall beat their swords into plowshares, and*

their spears into pruning hooks; nation shall not lift up sword against nation, neither shall they learn war anymore.

Christians understand that this comes about through the Messiah, the Prince of Peace.

Isaiah 9:6-7

⁶ *For to us a child is born, to us a son is given; and the government shall be upon his shoulder, and his name shall be called Wonderful Counselor, Mighty God, Everlasting Father, Prince of Peace.*

⁷*Of the increase of his government and of peace there will be no end, on the throne of David and over his kingdom, to establish it and to uphold it with justice and with righteousness from this time forth and forevermore. The zeal of the LORD of hosts will do this.*

Ephesians 2:14-21 (English Standard Version)

¹⁴*For he himself is our peace, who has made us both one and has broken down in his flesh the dividing wall of hostility* ¹⁵*by abolishing the law of commandments expressed in ordinances, that he might create in himself one new man in place of the two, so making peace,* ¹⁶*and might reconcile us both to God in one body through the cross, thereby killing the hostility.* ¹⁷*And he came and preached peace to you who were far off and peace to those who were near.* ¹⁸*For through him we both have access in one Spirit to the Father.* ¹⁹*So then you are no longer strangers and aliens, but you are fellow citizens with the saints and members of the household of God,* ²⁰ *built on the foundation of the apostles and prophets, Christ Jesus himself being the cornerstone,* ²¹ *in whom the whole structure, being joined together, grows into a holy temple in the Lord.*

So there is a unity intended by God, brought about through faith in Christ, which results in peace among humankind. There is even a specific Biblical understanding of the ongoing connection between Jews and Christians taught in the New Testament.

"For if you (Christians) were cut from what is by nature a wild olive tree, and grafted, contrary to nature, into a cultivated olive tree, how much more will these, the natural branches (Jews), be grafted back into their own olive tree." **(Romans 11:24)**

Together this new "tree" makes up "The Israel of God" (Gal. 6:16). The goal is reconciliation, unity, and love brought about by faith in Jesus Christ.

"By this all people will know that you are my disciples, if you have love for one another" (John 13:35).

Have Christians always exhibited this? No, of course not! But the Bible sets it forth as the correct perspective, and it has been demonstrated at different times and places, in spite of the "normal" sinful human tendency to abuse power over those not in one's "group." The Bible clearly teaches that there is an "organic" connection between the Jewish people and Christians, a connection which God will renew in His time. But the Bible is also quite plain about new revelations which contradict the Gospel. **"There are some,"** writes the Apostle Paul, **"who trouble you and want to distort the gospel of Christ. But even if we or an angel from heaven should preach to you a gospel contrary to the one we preached to you, let him be accursed. As we have said before, so now I say again: If anyone is preaching to you a gospel contrary to the one you received, let him be accursed"** (Galatians 1:7-9). Notice that the penalty for a false Gospel is spiritual, not political.

> "Significantly, while the West has for some time now lamented the Crusades as mistaken, there has never been any mention from any serious Islamic authority of regret for the centuries and centuries of jihad and dhimmitude perpetrated against other societies. But this is hardly surprising: while religious violence contradicts the fundamentals of Christianity, religious violence is written into Islam's DNA." (Gregory M. Davis "Islam 101" http://www.jihadwatch.org/islam-101.html)

By contrast to the peace and unity held up as a standard in the Bible, Islam's sacred texts make a virtue out of dominating *kafirs*, non-Muslims.

Where Muslims are in the ascendancy, it is the will of Allah that they should compel *kafirs* to submit. It is in this way that peace will come, when all have come into the House of Islam, whether by personal conviction or by force.

This is the hope Osama Bin Laden held out to Americans before the attacks of 9/11 in his letter where he said that "it is to this religion (Islam) that we call you; the seal of all the previous religions....It is the religion of showing kindness to others, establishing justice between them, granting them their rights, and defending the oppressed and the persecuted....It is the religion of Jihad in the way of Allah so that Allah's Word and religion reign Supreme."

Bin Laden can speak of "kindness" and "jihad" in the same letter. That's because kindness is to be shown to fellow-Muslims. If Americans accept Islam, that is how they will know kindness from people like Bin Laden. "Justice" means *sharia* law, which reflects the will of Allah for society. Islam supports "rights" — the rights of Muslims against all who would oppress or persecute them. For example, when Mohammed is featured in sarcastic cartoons, this is persecution of Muslims. When an obscure Florida pastor burns a copy of the Koran, this is oppression of Muslims. When France forbids women from completely covering their faces in public, this is oppression of Muslims. *Jihad* requires striving against such things. It also requires the destruction of Christian church buildings in predominantly Muslim communities. Bombing the church of a minority Christian group is *jihad*, because it protects the Muslim community against the oppression of having to look at something in their midst which is an offense to Allah. Sending rockets into civilian population centers of Israel is *jihad*, because it is driving out Jews whose very presence is supposedly offensive to Islam.

Such is the kind of thinking behind someone like Osama Bin Laden and others whom we call "radical" Muslims, or "Muslim terrorists," such as Hamas and Hezbollah. Fortunately not all Muslims follow through on the teachings of Islam to this extent. Unfortunately, though, there is a high respect in the Muslim world for people like Bin Laden because such people are perceived as being faithful to the revelation brought by Mohammed.

Many who would never do such violent acts themselves respect those who do them, because they do it in the cause of Allah, imitating the example of Mohammed. Also, many who do not commit violent acts give *zakat*, Islamic charity, to groups which do endorse and commit such acts.

Notice the difference between Christian and Muslim responses to atrocious behavior. When a Florida pastor publicly burned the Koran, many Christians cried out against such an act of disrespect. But the overwhelming majority of Palestinian Muslims support Hamas targeting Israeli civilians. So burning a sacred book is "evil," but killing people is "good." Large numbers of Muslims rioted when the Mohammed cartoons were published, and innocent Christians, including at least two nuns, were murdered. Large numbers of Muslims celebrated when the Twin Towers came down. What's the basis for the contrast between the response of the Christians and these multiple violent responses of Muslims? It's not that Christians are inherently better people than Muslims, or incapable of evil acts. It's that the Bible, the foundational text for Christianity, speaks so loudly against violence and disrespect toward other human beings, while the Koran, Hadith, and Sira all clearly proclaim that violence and disrespect toward *kafirs* is pleasing to Allah.

If you know the history and political doctrine of Islam, your perspective on what is happening today will change. You can see that Islam's history of killing over 270 million *kafirs* is simply continuing today. *Kafir* civilization is being attacked on a daily basis by Islam. When a Christian is persecuted, a *kafir* is persecuted. The way to halt this destruction begins with learning the facts about Islam, about the Koran, and about Mohammed, coupled with a willingness to communicate to others what you know.

QUESTIONS:

1. Mohammed claimed to be in the line of Jewish prophets. What are at least two things which suggest he was mistaken?

2. Give two or more examples of ways in which Islam is more than what we usually mean by "a religion."

Endnotes:

1   The reader is again referred to Bill Warner's detailed statistical analysis of Islamic texts at http://www.politicalislam.com/downloads/Statistical-Islam.pdf

2   Adapted in part from Bill Warner's _Thirteen Lessons on Political Islam_ Number 5 "'The Jews." May be downloaded from the Internet in its entirety at http://www.politicalislam. com/blog/category/thirteen-talks-on-political-islam/

3   Of great value on the roots of Islamic hatred of the Jews is Al-Yahud: Eternal Islamic Enmity and the Jews by E. Al-Maqdisi & Sam Solomon ANM Publishers Charlottesville, VA 2010.

4   Adapted in part from Bill Warner's _Thirteen Lessons on Political Islam_ Number 6 "'The Christians." May be downloaded from the Internet in its entirety at http://www.political islam.com/blog/category/thirteen-talks-on-political-islam/

5   See, for example, the critique offered by S. Solomon & E. Al-Maqdisi in The Common Word: the Undermining of the Church ANM Publishers, Charlottesville, VA 2009.

6   As one example, see the persecution described in Muslim Jihad in Christian Ethiopia: Lessons for the West in Appendix I

Chapter 4
The Submission of *Dhimmis* and Slaves

The Dhimmi[1]

A *Dhimmi* is someone who lives in fear of Islam but agrees not to resist political Islam, and will even support it in return for living safely. *Dhimmitude* is the attitude of mind of the dhimmi. Today we see our politicians, journalists and intellectuals play the role of dhimmis. The Dhimmi was a unique invention of Mohammed's. He created a new type of creature, a semi-slave. Dhimmis began with what Mohammed did to the Jews of Khaybar. He took their land and then let them work the land and as dhimmis pay a tax, the *jhizya*, that was half of their income.

A Dhimmi was a *kafir* who lived in an Islamic country. The first dhimmis were the Jews, but Christians and others were added later. Jews and Christians could still practice their religion, but privately. The laws were Islamic. Even what one could wear was dictated by Islamic law. Dhimmis were not really free. For instance, a church couldn't ring its bells because bells are a sign of Satan, according to Mohammed. A Dhimmi couldn't hold any job that made him a supervisor over Muslims. This limited rank in the military and promotions in business. If Christians wanted to repair the church, or Jews the synagogue, they had to get permission from the government, which meant churches and synagogues could fall into complete disrepair, with rain dripping on the worshippers. All of these laws established a second-class citizenship; the dhimmi did not have civil rights. A dhimmi couldn't sue a Muslim or prosecute a crime against a Muslim. This type of citizen had no power and had to pay the *jizya* tax, because the Koran says that the dhimmi must pay the *jizya*. Traditionally, when the Christian or the Jewish dhimmi came to pay their yearly jizya tax, they were humiliated-- grabbed by the beard, slapped in the face, or made to kneel and give the money. They were humiliated because the Koran said that dhimmis are to be humiliated.

Some Islamic countries, particularly when the country's ruler felt powerful, were more tolerant towards the dhimmis. A dhimmi could even rise to a decent level of power within government, but that could all vanish overnight. The treatment of the dhimmi was shown in Coptic Egypt. The Copts were the original Egyptians, and they were all Christians by the time Islam arose in the 600's AD. A dhimmi could have his tongue removed if he spoke the Coptic language in front of an Islamic government official. The dhimmi was always persecuted and was never really an equal.

When the Egyptian military tried to conquer the Byzantine Christians, but lost a battle, back in Egypt the Muslims rioted against the Christians, and Christians were killed. Riots were one of the favorite ways to punish the dhimmi. When Smyrna, the last of the seven churches of Asia spoken of in the book of Revelation, was destroyed in 1922, it was not done with the military and bulldozers. No, rioting Muslims did it. Riots are a form of jihad. The dhimmi could always be persecuted, not only in the courts of law, but a riot could destroy an entire section of a city. Dhimmis were killed if they criticized Mohammed, and actually dhimmis were not even supposed to study Mohammed at all.

There was a formal treaty called the Treaty of Omar (or "Umar," the second Caliph after Mohammed) which laid out everything that was to be done to the dhimmi. A dhimmi could not ride a horse, but he could ride a donkey. Dhimmis caught on a horse could be pulled off and beaten. When a dhimmi met a Muslim on the sidewalk, he had to step out into the street and let the Muslim pass. The dhimmi also had to wear special clothing or, if not special clothing, a belt or a patch on the clothing to immediately identify the wearer as a dhimmi. The only protection that a Christian or a Jew had would be to make Muslim friends because many times the Muslim friend could keep the full severity of dhimmi laws from his Christian or Jewish friend. Then as now there were Muslims who chose to show kindness to dhimmis regardless of what Islamic law prescribed.

The persecution of the dhimmis was unrelenting. It went on for generation after generation. Finally most dhimmis gave up and became Muslims. All of a sudden the new Muslim had more money because he didn't have to pay the Jhizya tax. Converted dhimmis could be promoted in their jobs. They would not be spit at or have stones thrown at them on the street. They could go to court and be treated as full, equal, citizens.

As the centuries passed, more and more dhimmis converted to Islam. Dhimmitude, which is the attitude of mind of the dhimmi, allows the destruction of the civilization into which Islam moves because the only way out is to become more Islamic, giving up all of one's old culture. When Islam moved into Coptic Egypt, the culture was a blend of the old culture of the Pharaohs mixed with the culture of the Greeks. But all of the Coptic culture eventually disappeared, except some of the church buildings that were permitted to remain, as were the pyramids, which were stripped of their beautiful marble veneer and the Sphinx's nose broken off. Why? Because Islam is a complete civilization, it cannot accommodate other civilizations within itself. Everything in Islam, including law and politics, is given by Allah through Mohammed, and thus any deviation is impermissible in the long run.

So, over time, Islam seeks to annihilate all other cultures by dhimmitude. The lack of civil rights, the abuse, humiliation, and tax burden wears away any resistance to becoming Islamic. People get new Islamic names and the names of cities change and then the former culture's history vanishes. Once a nation has been fully Islamicized, all of its history disappears. When Napoleon invaded Egypt, none of the Muslims there could explain anything about the old temples, the statues, or the pyramids. The people were ignorant of Egypt's history. They didn't know anything because the culture of the pharaohs had been annihilated. Only artifacts remained. The study of those artifacts by Egyptologists is how we've learned about ancient Egypt. The culture of the Greeks in Anatolia (now Turkey) was destroyed. In Pakistan, now a Muslim country, the native culture was Hindu. Afghanistan was a Buddhist culture that has been completely annihilated.

Part of the Islamic takeover and eradication of a nation and its culture is the destruction of sacred sites. Churches or temples that were beautiful or valuable were converted to mosques. One estimate has put the number of churches destroyed by the Islamic conquest of Turkey near 20,000, and some say more. India had magnificent temples of Hindu worship which the Muslims destroyed. Islam invented defacing. When Islam invaded a country, all of the religious objects were destroyed, following the example of Mohammed who had destroyed all religious art. If there was a mural on a wall, the face was destroyed. Once the face was gone, the rest of the object was left. That's why the Sphinx's nose had to go. The purpose of dhimmitude was twofold: (1) to bring in money by the dhimmi tax and (2) to slowly grind out the dhimmi's culture. This process worked really well. As a matter of fact, it was so successful that there is a black hole in history about dhimmitude. Virtually no one studies this part of world history. It is not taught in universities. In some divinity schools which consider themselves sophisticated the dhimmi is discussed. However, what is said is, "Oh, the dhimmi was protected." It makes life as a dhimmi sound warm and fuzzy, like living in the arms of your grandparents. And the question arises: protected from what and whom? What is not taught is how the dhimmi was humiliated. When it is said that the dhimmi was protected, it is quite true, up to a point. To be protected as a dhimmi meant that as long as one kept paying the tax he would not be killed nor would his goods be stolen, unless there was a riot. In a riot no dhimmi was protected.

Today there is no Islamic country strong enough to have full dhimmi status as a formal policy. However, both dhimmis and slavery are part of

Islam, and the doctrine of Islam cannot be changed. The Koran is complete, perfect and absolute. The condition and rule of the dhimmi is laid out in the Koran, so the dhimmi cannot be eliminated. The reason that there is not currently a formal dhimmi status is that Islam is not powerful enough to enforce it on a large scale. So instead of having a formal status for the dhimmi, bigotry and prejudice limit the civil rights of non-Muslims in Muslim-majority countries. This leads to various ongoing persecutions of *kafirs* in all Muslim-majority countries and in Muslim-majority regions of other countries. For example, many Islamic countries make it a capital crime to speak badly of Mohammed. So it is simple for a Muslim who wants to harm a *kafir* to accuse him of disrespecting Mohammed. Because the non-Muslim's word counts less in court testimony than the Muslim's, unless the *kafir* has Muslim friends who will speak on his behalf, he is going to jail, or even facing execution. This is a reality today in countries like Pakistan and Iran.

Today dhimmis are not just inside Islamic countries. Most *kafirs* all over the world are dhimmis in some measure, because they readily defer to Islam on all sorts of issues. *Kafirs* in places where Muslims are not the majority have replaced the dhimmi legal status with the mind of the dhimmi, an attitude known as dhimmitude. Let's look at some examples of dhimmitude. Soon after 9/11 this scene was repeated in many cities: a public gathering would be held and there would be a minister, a rabbi, and an Imam and someone to operate as Master of Ceremonies. At this gathering the rabbi and minister said that they all worshipped the same god as the Muslims. But if the Christian minister was asked, "Have you read the Koran? Do you know the traditions? Do you know the Sira (the life of Mohammed)?" The Minister normally would answer, "Well, no." Then the rabbi would be asked, "Have you read the Koran?" "No." "Do you know the life of Mohammed?" "No." "Have you read the traditions?" "No." Then the Imam was asked, "Have you read the New Testament?" "Oh, yes!" "Have you read the Old Testament?" "Sure!"

There is something wrong with this picture, because the Rabbi and the Minister said, "Oh, we worship the same God," but then said, "Well we really don't know anything about Allah or Islam." So why then did they say they worshipped the same god as Islam? This is an attempt to please the Muslims even though it means telling a lie, which is an example of dhimmitude. Think about it--religious leaders standing up in public and telling a deliberate lie! Why? Because it sounds good and because inside nearly every Christian, every Jew, and for that matter nearly every *kafir* is a timidity or even a fear of Islam. Added to that today we have "political correctness," saying that minority groups can never be talked about in a negative way. For some reason 1.7 billion Muslims are categorized as a minority with delicate feelings, while in countries where Christians are clearly a minority, like modern Britain, "political correctness" has no scruples about denigrating Christianity, or abridging the rights of Christians to practice their faith. For example, there are hospitals in Britain that have prayer rooms for Muslims, but forbid Christian nurses from wearing a cross around their necks because the cross is offensive to Islam. This is dhimmitude.

Dhimmitude is the attitude of one who always tries to placate the bully. Islam is always pressuring for this attitude of submission. This pressure is a form of jihad, and as we've seen, jihad in order to produce Islam, submission, is what Islam requires of Muslims. For example, *Sharia*, Muslim Law, permits a Muslim to have up to four wives. In the West we have laws requiring monogamy. However, Britain allows a Muslim to bring in more than one wife, and they all can qualify for welfare. This again is dhimmitude. Dhimmitude is submitting to Islam because submitting seems safe and easy.

We see dhimmitude in government hiring and promotion. Government agencies give preference to Muslim Arabs over Christian Arabs in translation work. Government workers are treated to forums where Muslims come in and talk about Islam, but Buddhists do not get a forum to explain Buddhism, nor Hindus a forum to explain Hinduism. And of course Christians would never get a forum to explain Christianity, nor Jews a forum to explain Judaism. That would violate the separation of Church and State! But, for some reason, Islam is treated differently. This is Dhimmitude.

In another form of Dhimmitude, our universities do not teach the history of the Dhimmi nor do they teach the history of Islamic conquest. The universities teach a history of Islam which is one of glorious triumph but in which for some mysterious reason no injustice or suffering ever occurred.

The United States prides itself on freedom of the press and political speech. Citizens are supposed to have the right to stand up and say anything about politics. People might laugh at you, and they may not vote for you, but it's not a crime to speak. But remember the Mohammed cartoons? No newspaper in the United States published the Mohammed cartoons. Mohammed was a political figure and yet our newspapers, by law having freedom of the press, did not publish those cartoons. Newspapers defended themselves by saying that they did not want to offend anyone, but some of the same newpapers had previously published photos of a crucifix submerged in urine. Politics frequently involves offending someone. Newspapers are in the business of offending people at times. So it is reasonable to conclude that the newspapers' real reason was not that they actually never want to offend anyone, but because dhimmis are always afraid of Islam. Dhimmis are always looking for a way to placate and appease. When the cartoons were not shown on TV nor published in the newspapers, those refusals to exercise freedom of speech or freedom of the press were acts of dhimmis. Their motive was not being nice; they were being dhimmis, otherwise they would be equally nice to other religions.

To slowly accept Sharia Law is another form of dhimmitude. Airports in the United States are changing the plumbing so that Muslims will have a place to wash their feet before prayer. Universities have "meditation rooms," however, the Muslims monopolize them. If a university is questioned about this seemingly unfair use, it will not intervene on behalf of non-Muslim students. That is dhimmitude. When a workplace that runs an assembly line says, "If you're Muslim we will provide for you a place to pray, and you can leave the production line when it is prayer time," that's dhimmitude. Why? because the employer does not provide that opportunity for any other employee. It is the dhimmi who operates out of fear in order to placate Islam.

In the United States and in Europe there is no formal Dhimmi status, but there is dhimmitude. As a result of this attitude, Europe is rapidly becoming Islamicized. Unless there is a radical change of direction, the day will come when the churches in Europe live in fear, as they do now in Turkey or Egypt or Syria or Lebanon. Churches will have to get permission from the Muslims who are controlling the local political process to get the roof fixed. The reason people will be subject to Islamic rule is that they never studied the history of the political Islam and learned about the fate of dhimmis. Any people who do not study the history of political Islam and study the history of the dhimmi and learn from it are doomed to repeat the subjection of the dhimmis, lose their political rights, and ultimately lose their civilization.

Slavery[2]

You do not know the history of slavery if you do not know about Islam and slavery. Slavery is a very important part of a highly developed doctrine in Islam. It has a 1400-year-old history which is still alive today in Africa. Mohammed was a slaver who dealt in every aspect of slavery. It is impossible to study the history of Mohammed and the beginnings of Islam and avoid the role of slavery. The politically correct version of slavery is that it only happened when white men showed up in wooden ships off the coast of Africa, went into the bush, captured slaves and brought them back to sell in America. That is the generally accepted history of slavery in America. This does contain a part of the truth but it is not remotely the story of world slavery, or even the history of slave trading in the Americas. To study slavery worldwide, you must study Islam because Islam has enslaved all others: Africans, Europeans, and Asians. Wherever Islam has gone it has enslaved everybody without discrimination..

Francis Bok, a Christian from Sudan, appeared at a university to give a talk a few years ago. It was very interesting because he was an actual freed African slave. He and his sister had gone to the market to sell beans and while they were in the market place, Muslim jihadis showed up. They captured his sister and him along with others and set out on a forced march. Every night his sister was raped by the members of the troop. When they finally got to the jihadis' camp, they were put on the block and sold as slaves. Once Francis was sold, he was taken to the new master's home. He was placed in the center of the family and every member of the family took a small stick and began to beat him with it. Then they informed him that he no longer had any name. From this day forward there was no more Francis Bok. From now on he was only "Abd." "Abd" is the word for a black slave. Abd is an Arabic word, but it's only one of about forty different words that Islam has for a slave. In English we simply have one word — slave, so why would the Arabic language have so many words for slave? Abd means both "black slave" and "an African." In other words, in Arabic, African = black slave.

There's an Arabic word for white slave-mamluk. There's a word for a Hindu slave. Perhaps you're beginning to grasp the idea that over a long period of time Arabs have had a lot to do with the slave trade. Languages don't change overnight. It took a long time to accumulate 40 different words for different kinds of slaves.

Francis Bok, now a non-person, the slave "Abd," was given a room with the animals in the barn. They gave him some straw to lie on. Francis Bok and other living survivors of slavery are important because when slavery is brought up to Muslims they admit that it happened in the past but insist that it no longer happens. And anyway, they say, Muslims treated their slaves really well. Perhaps that message was not given to Francis Bok's masters because in the 1980's and 1990's he was required to sleep in the barn with animals. He tried to escape, but was captured and beaten.

By the way, as soon as he escaped the Arabic language had a new word for him. The Arabic language has a word for an escaped male slave. It has a word for an escaped female slave. And it has a word for an escaped child slave. The Arabic language since the rise of Islam has put a fine point on slavery.

Francis kept working and plotting and growing a little older and a little stronger. Finally he found an opportune time and he escaped and he set out on his own forced march, this time not a forced march to slavery but a forced march to freedom. He got first to Egypt and finally to America where he works with an organization called The American Anti-Slavery Group, (www.iabolish.org). It was this group that sponsored him to speak at the university.

Francis was asked from the audience "Who captured you?" And he said "Muslims". Then later someone said, "Muslims can react very violently, indeed they can kill you if they don't like what you say about them. Are you afraid for your own life in saying that Muslims captured and enslaved you?" His remark was memorable. He said, "I am now a free man. Now I can die because I will die as a free man." Think about that. "I will die as a free man." You can learn more about Francis Bok by searching the Internet under his name.

Now let's stop and take a closer look at the white man's involvement with slavery. Did he show up on the coast of Africa in a wooden ship to get slaves? Yes he did. But he didn't go into the bush to get them. He went to the slave market where he bought them at a wholesale price in wholesale lots. Bills of sale, money, and invoices were exchanged. He left with his boatload of slaves that he got from the Muslim slave trader. The Muslims had been trading slaves and capturing slaves in Africa for some 900 years. The white man just represented a new market. Muslims had been enslaving before the white man and so when white people put together new laws that eliminated slavery and the slave trade, Muslims just kept on with their old business. They are not inhibited by the laws of the kafir.

We know that Mohammed had black slaves. It says so in the Hadith. It says so in the Sira. So slavery is nothing new to Islam. In fact, slavery is a type of the ideal in Islam. The ideal Muslim is the slave of Allah and indeed Mohammed called himself the slave of Allah because inside of Islam there is no freedom.

Can we contrast this with one of the Bible's famous verses? **"For freedom Christ has set us free; stand firm therefore, and do not submit again to a yoke of slavery"** (Galatians 5:1). Christ brings complete freedom from the requirements of becoming righteous by obeying the Law. Yet there is indeed a Biblical encouragement to be a *doulos*, the Greek for "servant" or "slave." Here is an example from the same Apostle Paul who wrote Galatians 5:1.

> ³*Do nothing from rivalry or conceit, but in humility count others more significant than yourselves.* ⁴*Let each of you look not only to his own interests, but also to the interests of others.* ⁵ *Have this mind among yourselves, which is yours in Christ Jesus,* ⁶ *who, though he was in the form of God, did not count equality with God a thing to be grasped,* ⁷*but made himself nothing, taking the form of a servant, being born in the likeness of men.* ⁸*And being found in human form, he humbled himself by becoming obedient to the point of death, even death on a cross.* (Philippians 2:3-8).

So Christian "slavery" is in imitation of Christ, and means promoting the interests of others before oneself. Christians can do this freely because they are not under the bondage of having to produce their own right standing with God. The same grace from God that brings freedom from legalistic bondage also allows us to willingly serve God by serving each other.

But to be a Muslim is to be a "slave of Allah," following all the rules given in the Koran and in the Sunna of Mohammed. The "Sunna," remember, is the term for the Hadith and Sira combined. A slave who is under complete submission to a master is thus a picture of the ideal Muslim.

Islam has enslaved many peoples, including Europeans. It's estimated that a total of 25 million Africans have been sold as slaves and that about a million Europeans have been sold into slavery. Indeed, the one word that we have in English for slave comes from the Slavic people, the Slavs. The Muslims took many slaves out of Eastern Europe and the primary ethnic group they preyed upon were the Slavs, so we adopted the term "slave" from the Slavs who were being dragged off as slaves by Muslim conquerors.

Historically in Islam, there have been different uses for different races of people as slaves. The Black Africans were usually put into rough, hard work and frequently died at it. It was a death sentence to be a Black slave in the Saharan salt mines, for example. Whites were usually put to work in what we would call "white collar" jobs. They could even become leaders in the Army. The highest priced slave in the Meccan slave market for 1400 years never changed. It was always a white woman who brought the highest price. Writings from Medieval Islamic documents show that Muslims then were very free and open in discussing which race was used for which job. For instance the white woman was preferred as a slave of pleasure, but if you could not afford her since she was the most expensive, then an Ethiopian woman was the second best choice.

This preference for white women as sexual slaves was, like everything in Islam, put in place by Mohammed. You see, Mohammed had all manner of slaves, but his favorite sexual partner was a white woman. Her name was Miriam, or Mary. She was a Coptic Christian. Well, since the Koran says more than 70 times to follow the example of Mohammed, this means that the preference of all Muslims who wish a slave for sexual pleasure is the same as Mohammed, a white slave. So the Sunnah, the example, of Mohammed is appalling if you are a white woman.

There is an interesting special kind of slave that was used in Islam, that of the Eunuch. Generally these were male Black slaves and the castration process removed all the sexual organs. Eunuchs are even referred to in the Koran because they can see the woman of the house unveiled. The Koran is very clear about slavery. It's quite desirable and it has only one limitation, you cannot enslave Muslims. Only kafirs can be enslaved and poor Francis Bok, being a Christian, was a kafir.

In Francis's case, he ran away to get his freedom, but he might have escaped being a slave if he had chosen to become a slave of Allah, a Muslim. The rules of slavery inside of Islam, and there are many rules, is that it is good to free slaves because that brings a great merit with Allah, but you don't free a kafir slave. So perhaps Francis could have converted to Islam and been freed through that path. But Francis Bok wanted to be a Christian. He did not want to be a Muslim, so he had to take the only path open to him, which was flight.

The full history of slavery is not taught in any university in the United States. Nor is it easy to find books written that include the fact of Islam's role in world slavery. The only accepted history of slavery is the 250 years that Europeans and Americans practiced it against black Africans. Yet it also was first Europeans, then Americans, who did the most to stop the international slave trade. It began with evangelical Christian William Wilberforce's leadership in the British Parliament passing laws requiring the British Navy to intercept slave ships. This eventually-successful interdiction of slave shipping, however, did not end Islamic enslavement of Africans. Out of the 25 million slaves that were taken out of Africa, 11 million were sold in the Americas. The other 14 million were sold in the Islamic regions of West and North Africa and in Islamic parts of Asia.

There was an additional side effect of slavery. For every slave captured, the slavers had to kill others. For instance, Francis Bok's parents were killed. The slavers showed up with armed troops, and killed all those who tried to defend their tribe or village. When the slavers finally killed all the defenders, they could then take the best of the survivors as slaves. The old, the sick, and the very young were left behind, because they couldn't survive the forced march that comes right after capture. Estimates of the collateral damage from taking one slave vary. Some of those who visited Africa during the peak slave trading days reported that as many as ten had to die to produce one slave in the wholesale market. Others said no, only five. So using the lower figure we can see that out of the 25 million enslaved, there were over 100 million Africans, perhaps 120 million Africans or more, who have died over a 1400 year period up to and including today. When you hear about "Darfur" in Sudan in the news, the genocide there includes slave-taking, but this is never mentioned, and these appalling figures for the Islamic enslaving of black Africans never get talked about.

Now then, let's talk about Mohammed's role in slavery. As mentioned before, the biography of Mohammed, the Sira, and the Hadith, his recorded sayings, are full of details about his life. He had slaves in his family. His first wife, Khadijah, owned slaves. Indeed, one of Mohammed's first converts was a black slave and Mohammed himself owned black slaves. Mohammed was deep into slavery. As a matter of fact, slavery was one of the chief ways he financed Jihad. He was involved in having kafir men killed so their women and children could be made slaves. He sent his own jihadists out on slave missions. He gave away slaves as gifts.

He owned all kinds of slaves including males and females, both black and white. He passed around slaves for the purpose of the sexual pleasure of his companions, the men who were his chief lieutenants. He stood by and prayed while others beat slaves. He participated in the rape of female captives after conquest, whose status was automatically that of "slave." He captured slaves and wholesaled them to raise money for Jihad. One of his favorite sexual partners was a slave who bore him a son. He got slaves as gifts from other rulers. The very pulpit he preached from was made by a slave. Some of his cooks were slaves. He was treated medically by a slave. He had a slave tailor. He declared that any slave who ran away from his master would not have his prayers answered. Happily, he was wrong about that for Francis Bok because he did escape from slavery. His prayers were answered because his prayers were to be free.

It is interesting to note how slavery falls into line with Islam's two fundamental principles: submission and duality. Submission, because who is more submissive than a slave? And duality, because Islamic doctrine creates a separate legal and ethical classification for the slave. So it's no wonder that for all these years Islam has been involved in slavery. Allah wants slaves and Allah wants Muslims to enslave others, because after you keep them as a slave long enough, they will convert to Islam and if they don't, then their children will. The Koran and Islam see slavery as a great good, because it brings about submission to Islam and to Allah's prophet Mohammed.

Now you may be saying to yourself, "If it's in the Koran, do they still do it?" In fact, Muslims are still involved in slavery. You've just learned about Francis Bok's story, but there are many other examples. For example, women who are brought in from the Philippines to work in Saudi Arabia are often treated as slaves. Their passports are taken away and they may or may not get back home. Slavery is in the Koran, and it's in the Sunna. The more Islam controls a society, the more slavery rears its head. So it is still fairly evident in Saudi Arabia, Brunei, and northern Sudan, but is kept quieter in other places, although still practiced. Slavery cannot be removed from Islamic doctrine because, unlike our constitution, Islamic doctrine is eternal. It's permanent. It's forever.

Here is a quote from an internet article published May 23, 2011.

A well known Islamic leader in Egypt by the name of Abu Ishak Al Huweini, who often appears on Egyptian TV, has recently said the following in Arabic and I have translated it into English:

> "We are at a time of Jihad; Jihad for the sake of Allah is a pleasure, a true pleasure. Mohammed's followers used to compete to do it. The reason we are poor now is because we have abandoned jihad. If only we can conduct a jihadist invasion at least once a year or if possible twice or three times, then many people on Earth would become Muslims. And if anyone prevents our dawa or stands in our way, then we must kill them <u>or take as hostage and confiscate their wealth, women and children. Such battles will fill the pockets of the Mujahid who can return home with 3 or 4 slaves, 3 or 4 women and 3 or 4 children. This can be a profitable business</u> if you multiply each head by 300 or 400 dirham. This can be like financial shelter whereby a jihadist, in time of financial need, can always sell one of these heads (meaning slavery). No one can make that much money in one deal (from hard work) even if a Muslim goes to the West to work or do trade. In time of need, that is a good resource for profit."
>
> *Nonie Darwish, "Solving Poverty — the Islamic Way"* <u>www.frontpagemag.com</u> 05/23/11, <u>http://frontpagemag.com/2011/05/23/solving-poverty-the-islamic-way/</u> ?utm_source=Front Page+Magazine&utm_medium=email&utm_campaign=38639add4c-RSS_EMAIL_CAMPAIGN

When the famous missionary explorer David Livingston was in Africa he saw the slave trade up close. He said that the paddle wheels on the boat he was on frequently hit slaves who had drowned in the river or the bodies of those who were killed in the process of trying to get slaves or fight slavers. He described a peculiar disease among slaves that the slave owners told him about. "The strangest disease I have seen in this country really seems to be broken heartedness and it attacks *kafirs* who have been captured and made slaves. Speaking with many who later died from it, they ascribe that their only pain was to the heart and place the hand correctly on that spot. Some slavers expressed surprise to me that these men would die seeing that they had plenty to eat and no work. It really seems that they died of a broken heart." He spoke with slave traders a long time about what they did and the Muslims told him that their object in capturing slaves was to get them into their possession and make them become Muslims.

This history is deeply sad, but the saddest thing is that it's not taught. Our universities don't teach it. The universities don't even teach how white people were also enslaved or how many Hindus were sold into slavery. We must teach the complete history of slavery in our schools and universities. Only then can we fully understand this dreadful history.

Not only that, but while rightly condemning European and American complicity in slavery for 250 years, it should be brought out that it was countries with Christianity in their history that moved to outlaw slavery in the territories they controlled. Islamic governments have never acted to outlaw slavery. They can't, because slavery is a part of the Koran, Hadith, and Sira.

Every Muslim is a slave of Allah. Slavery is Islam's dark secret. Islam has enslaved Europeans, Africans and Asians. Unfortunately, Western intellectuals seem happy to cover up Islam's crimes against humanity. Dhimmitude again.

QUESTIONS:

1. It's suggested in this chapter that "dhimmitude" happens in part because the facts of Islamic conquest are so dreadful. Can you think of other reasons why many people today resist learning the facts about Islamic conquest?

2. Slavery appears in the Bible, but it was Christians in Britain who took the lead in opposing slavery. What Biblical basis did they have to do so?

Endnotes:

1   Adapted in part from Bill Warner's *Thirteen Lessons on Political Islam* Number 7 "'The Dhimmi." May be downloaded from the Internet in its entirety at http://www.political islam.com/blog/category/thirteen-talks-on-political-islam/

2   Adapted in part from Bill Warner's *Thirteen Lessons on Political Islam* Number 9 "'Slavery." May be downloaded from the Internet in its entirety at http://www.politicalislam.com/blog/category/thirteen-talks-on-political-islam/

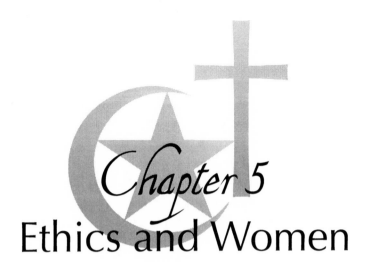

Chapter 5
Ethics and Women

Ethics[1]

If you can only know one thing about Islam, the most important is Islamic ethics. Islamic ethics do not share anything with ethics based on the Bible. Islamic ethics are dualistic. They have one set of rules for Muslims and another set of rules for everyone else, the *kafirs*. Kafirs can be deceived, robbed, murdered and raped, and as was explained in Chapter 2, there is even a word for sacred deceit which is used to bring kafirs into submission. As we go on, we will also see that ethical duality is also present among Muslims, for within Islam there is one set of rules for men and another for women. In the area of religion per se, the "Five Pillars," the rules for men and women are basically the same. But in the areas of marriage, family life, law, and politics, there are two different sets of rules for men and women.

Ethics is the great divide between Islam and all other cultures, but before we look at Islamic ethics, let's look at the basis for ethics in what we call "the West." Our ethics are based upon the Bible, especially upon the Golden Rule, namely, treat others as you would be treated. Who are the "others" in Biblical ethics? The others are ALL others, all other human beings. There's no elimination of someone because of race, sex, ethnicity, or religion. This comes from the Biblical perspective that all human beings are made in God's image, and thus are objects of His love. We are to mirror God's love for all human beings in our relations with all those whom God loves. This has had wider application. For instance, in our politics everyone is to be treated fairly and equally before the law. Political systems without a Biblical foundation always end with "some animals are more equal than others," in George Orwell's famous phrase from <u>Animal Farm</u>. Soviet communism, supposedly committed to equality, was a demonstration of this. Only the Golden Rule successfully frames the concepts of what we call "fair" or "just" and what we call "equal." Someone may jump up and say, "But we don't follow it all the time do we?" Here's what's important. No, it is true that we do not follow the Golden Rule all the time, either as individuals or as a society, because every person is pulled between two contradictory ideas. One idea is to treat others as I would like to be treated. The other very human idea is purely selfish and wants to look only to ourselves. When we focus on our own personal needs so much that we start harming or neglecting others, we can be corrected and brought back because our behavior is not based upon the Golden Rule. The Golden Rule lies behind both our ethical and our legal system. By the way, this shows how foolish it is to say, as some do, that "we don't want to legislate morality." Any law will always be based on some ethical principle. It's just a question of what principle: the Golden Rule? Or "might makes right"? Or, "just do what you feel"? Or, as in Islam, ethical duality.

Islam does not follow the Golden Rule. Indeed Islam explicitly denies the Golden Rule. The Koran never views humanity as a whole entity. Instead, humanity is always divided into the kafir and the Muslim. The Koran is very clear that the kafir is to be treated differently from the Muslim and this treatment can even be very violent. So this division into kafir and Muslim eliminates the possibility of having a Golden Rule. Islam's ethics therefore are unavoidably dualistic. It has one set of rules for those within Islam and another set of rules for the kafir. There is no such thing as a common humanity.

In Christianity there is certainly a conviction that those outside faith in Christ will be eternally lost. But this makes them the target of persuasion, not of political persecution or violence. Where "conversions" in the past have come about due to violence and political pressure, as in the medieval history of Lithuania, Christians now look back on such tactics as an abysmal failure to follow Christ. But political pressure and violence follows precisely the Sunna of Mohammed, and so it cannot be repudiated.

There is a famous verse in the Koran which says "there shall be no compulsion in religion" (la ikraha fi d-dini), al-Baqarah 2:256; al-Kahf 18:29; al-Ghashiyah 88:21-22.

This verse is one of the many said to be abrogated by the "sword verse" ayat al-sayf (at-taubah 9:5):

> "Then, when the sacred months have passed, slay the idolaters wherever ye find them, and take them (captive), and besiege them, and prepare for them each ambush. But if they repent and establish worship and pay the poor-due, then leave their way free. Lo! Allah is Forgiving, Merciful."

The last part of the verse: "But if they repent and establish worship and pay the poor-due, then leave their way free." means that if the kafirs become Muslims (with Islamic worship, particularly the confession of faith, the shahada, and the Islamic prayer, salat, and the payment of the Islamic alms, zakat), then the Muslims should not continue with killing them, but let them go.

The following hadith reinforces this.

> Narrated Abu Huraira:
> The Verse: "You (true Muslims) are the best of peoples ever raised up for mankind." means, the best of peoples for the people, as you bring them with chains on their necks till they embrace Islam. (Sahih Bukhari 6.80)

The other difference between Islamic ethics and Biblical ethics is that there is no fundamental concept of right and wrong in Islam. All ethics in Islam are based upon what Mohammed did and did not do, therefore Islamic ethics does not deal in the concepts of "right" and "wrong" but what is permitted and what is forbidden (*haram*). Mohammed is viewed as the perfect ethical pattern, because Allah in the Koran says that he is. Every Muslim is to follow him and do what he did and say what he said. The ethics of Islam are determined by what Mohammed did and said, his Sunnah, and by what the Koran says.

Let us examine Islamic ethics through the specific example of deceit. You'll remember from the second chapter that an important distinction between Yahweh, the LORD God of the Bible, and Allah is that Allah reveals himself as a superior deceiver, the best deceiver. In light of this, let's read some statements by contemporary Muslim leaders. Here is a quote from Ali Al Timimi, an internationally known Muslim scholar and imam who had U.S. government clearance. He even worked with a former White House Chief of Staff and was invited to speak to the U.S. military about Islam. Publicly this imam denounced Islamic violence and said: "My position against terrorism and Muslim-inspired violence against innocent people is well known by Muslims." This way of putting the matter is very clever. To most Americans, it sounds as though this imam is opposed to violence. But He does not say this exactly, he says "my position is well known by Muslims." This wording does not tell us honestly what his position is. So it is no surprise that privately another picture emerged of this imam. Five days after the attacks on September 11th he called them legitimate in his mosque and rallied young Muslim men there to carry out more Holy War and violent Jihad.

Another Islamic leader in this country, Abdurahman Alamoudi, who developed the Pentagon's Muslim chaplain corps and acted as a good will ambassador for our State Department, also denounced terror. "We are against all forms of terrorism" he claimed. "Our religion is against terrorism." But privately he raised major funds for Al-Qaeda and was caught on tape grumbling that Osama bin Laden had not killed enough kafirs in the U.S. Embassy bombings that preceded 9/11.

In our culture we would call these men liars. But this ethic does not apply inside Islamic ethics because what these men were practicing was intentional technical deceit of unbelievers in order to advance Islam. They were talking to kafirs when they said those things, so this was not lying in any sinful sense at all. Let's see what Mohammed said about deceiving the kafir.

In Medina there was a Jew named al-Ashraf. Al-Ashraf wrote a poem in which he condemned Mohammed and Mohammed at the mosque asked: "Who will rid me of Ashraf, the enemy of Allah and his prophet?" One of the Muslims said he would but a few days later Mohammed noticed that the task of killing al-Ashraf had not been done so he went to the man and said "What are you doing?" The man said, "Mohammed, in order to kill Ashraf I will have to tell a lie". Then Mohammed said, "Say whatever you need to say."

The Muslim took a couple of his friends and went to al-Ashraf and said they were getting sick and tired of Mohammed, but before they could leave, they needed to have a little money and were wondering if al Ashraf could help. They wanted to borrow some money. Al Ashraf said he would need some collateral to loan them money. And so they suggested that perhaps they could bring him their weapons — their swords and knives — and leave them in pawn. He agreed. So the next night the three Muslims showed up, their weapons in hand. But al-Ashraf was not concerned. They had come to pawn the weapons. They chatted with him in a friendly way and said, " it is night, a pleasant night, let us go for a walk and discuss things". So they did. But in the middle of the walk after they had recited some poetry, one of them grabbed him by the hair of the head, said to the other, "kill him", and they knifed him in the stomach and killed al-Ashraf.

When they came back to Mohammed, Mohammed was delighted at the death of the enemy of Allah and his prophet. He had given them permission to lie because they were dealing with a kafir and the lie advanced Islam. Here we have ethical duality. A Muslim is told not to lie to another Muslim, but with a kafir there is an option. The Muslim can tell the kafir the truth or he can tell him a lie if it will advance Islam. This was repeated many times in Mohammed's life. So much so that at one point he said, "Jihad is deceit."

Now let's go back to the statements of Muslim leaders that Islam does not use terror. And let's take another story. This one happened in Russia in Beslan, where there was a school with roughly a thousand people in it including the children and the staff. Some Muslim Jihadists attacked the school and took it over and held everyone in it. The Jihadists took all of the children and put them in the gymnasium. They were kept there for days without food or water. Finally the Russian special forces decided that they needed to go in. There was chaos, and as the children jumped out the windows and ran for safety, the Jihadists shot them in the back.

The attack continued. Once it became clear that they were going to lose the building the Jihadists fell back on their original plan. They had brought explosives and placed them in such a way that when they detonated them, the roof fell in on the children. This was the way that most of the children were killed. This was a terrible attack, but what happened after the attack illustrates Islam's ethical duality.

Muslim scholars and Muslim imams all said the same thing, "That was not Islam. In Islam we are forbidden to kill women and children." And that is true, there are Hadith which state that women and children are not to be killed. However, there are other Hadith in which Mohammed is getting ready to attack a tribe and the reason they're attacking is that these people are kafirs, not that they had done anything wrong. They decide to attack at night and they ask Mohammed: "What if we make a mistake in the dark and wind up killing women and children?" Mohammed answers, "They are from them (i.e. from the kafirs)."

Well now we have a contradiction. We have Mohammed saying "Do not kill women and children" and we have Mohammed saying "Kill them, they are from them." This is ethical duality. We have contradictory statements, but both of them are accepted as true. So jihadists can choose whichever they want and the jihadists in Beslan chose to kill the children. Why? "They are from them." That is, they are kafirs. In Mohammed's time, in which he developed the ethics of jihad, he always succeeded in keeping the kafirs confused. The Arabs, just like everyone else, had rules for warfare. Since Mohammed was an Arab they kept expecting him to follow the rules, but Mohammed did not follow the rules. He made them up as he went.

So far as terror not being Islamic, Mohammed said in one of the most famous Hadiths, "I have been given five things that have never been given to anyone before me." One of these things that he was given was that Allah allowed him to spread Islam by awe and terror. Mohammed embraced terror, so jihad includes terror. This means that when Muslim scholars say terror is not the way of Islam, they are practicing deceit. Remember, sacred deceit even has a special name in Arabic, *taqqyia*. To even have a concept of "sacred deceit" reveals a unique kind of ethics.

Here's another example of deceit in jihad. In modern times we have grown used to the fact that a Muslim jihadist can strap on dynamite and walk into a room filled with people, kafirs, and kill himself and everyone else. Muslim clerics after the fact say such behavior is not Islam because suicide is forbidden in Islam, and this is true. Suicide is forbidden in Islam. But there is a very famous Hadith in which Mohammed said that killing yourself while trying to kill kafirs sends you straight to heaven, therefore the ethical expectation of the person who kills himself in the face of killing others, if the others are kafirs, is that he will go straight to heaven. He is a martyr.

In the very term martyr in Islam, we see the distance between the Christian concept of "martyr," and Islam. In Christian terminology, "martyr," a Greek word meaning "witness," is someone whose life is taken from them because they remained faithful to Christ and the Gospel. Their death becomes a permanent testimony to the truth of what they believed. But the word "martyr" in Islam means someone who dies while making war on kafirs in the name of Allah.

Here's another example of the ethical divide. Currently in America there is debate over whether water boarding is torture, and what constitutes torture gets talked about in the media. There is, however, no debate inside the Islamic world about torturing kafirs, for the simple reason that Mohammed tortured kafirs. There's a famous story of a time when he attacked a tribe of Jews. After the Jews had surrendered, the victorious Muslims took the leader of the Jews and staked him out on the ground at Mohammed's orders. The reason they did this was they knew that the Jews had a buried treasure. Mohammed had a small fire built on the old man's chest but he would not speak. He would not give up the secret of the treasure so finally Mohammed said to cut him loose and he took him over to a jihadist who had lost his brother in the attack on the Jews and gave him the pleasure of killing the leader of the Jews. As a consequence, inside Islam there are no questions about whether torture can be used against kafirs. It is Sunna. It is the way of Mohammed to torture the kafir.

Islamic ethics are clearly laid out in the Hadith. Here are some statements about Islamic ethics found in various traditions. A Muslim is to never cheat another Muslim in business. A Muslim does not lie to another Muslim. A Muslim does not kill another Muslim. A Muslim does not bother another Muslim's wife. These statements are very dualistic because this behavior is only reserved for other Muslims. A Muslim is a brother to other Muslims. Anyone who knows Muslims says "wait a minute, I know a lot of Muslims and they don't lie to me and they don't cheat me in business. They don't come to work with dynamite and kill themselves and other people." This is quite true, and it again illustrates ethical duality. There are two ways to treat the kafir. He can be treated well, and the Golden Rule can even be applied to him if it will advance Islam, but the truth of how Islam views the kafir does not need to be told. The truth can be shaded. The most common form of this deceit is for Muslims to only discuss the Koran of Mecca. Only talking about the Koran of Mecca is telling a half-truth, not telling the whole truth. Again, although it's been said before, it bears repeating that many Muslims know only the religious aspect of Islam. However, leading spokesmen for Islam invariably know the whole truth of what the Koran and the Sunna of Mohammed teach, but they deny it because they know to publicly admit it puts Islam in a bad light.

In our courts, we "swear to tell the whole truth and nothing but the truth." "Nothing but the truth" prohibits direct lies. But it's equally important to "tell the whole truth" because telling half a truth is just another form of a lie. So when a Muslim will only discuss with a kafir the Koran of Mecca, the nicer half of the Koran, this is a form of deceit

Islamic ethics support how Muslims treat women. For instance, women can be beaten. Women are set apart in their own separate code. We'll look at this in more detail in a moment. There is also an ethical system for slavery, as covered in the last chapter. Mohammed was the perfect slave master. His Sunna laid out all the ways that slaves are to be treated. There is an ethical system for the treatment of the dhimmi, that strange political creature who is not quite a slave, but certainly not a full citizen.

So Islamic ethics lie behind everything that a Muslim is supposed to do, but this raises political questions. If a Muslim does not have to tell the kafir the truth, why would we use Muslim translators for Arabic documents inside the FBI and the CIA? Muslim translators take an oath, but Islam has a very unique interpretation of oaths, that is, an oath can always be changed by a Muslim for something better, and there is a Hadith which explicitly states this. But the Hadith does not really say what is better. That is the choice of the Muslim. So if we have a Muslim policeman or a military man who takes an oath to serve and protect, he can change it anytime he wishes. This is apparently what happened to Major Nidal Hasan, the Fort Hood assassin. And for that matter, this same changing of oaths is applied to treaties, including political treaties between governments. If the Muslim nation signs a treaty with a kafir government it can be abrogated at any time as long as Islam comes out on top.

To deal with Islam, it is critical that we understand its ethics. We individually, and our political leaders, assume that their ethics are the same as ours, but this assumption is based upon ignorance. Islamic ethics are quite different. Our ethics are based on the unitary principle of treating all people the same. The same rule applies to everyone. Islamic ethics are based upon having one set of ethics for believers and another set of ethics for kafirs. The ethical thing is to treat them differently. One cannot understand Islam without understanding its ethical duality. Even within Islam there is ethical duality in how men and women are treated. We'll take a look at this now.

Chapter 5: *Ethics and Women*   89

Women in Islam[2]

The dualism of Islam allows for two ways to treat women. They can be honored and protected or they can be beaten or otherwise mistreated. Today Western nations allow Islamic women to be treated as Islam wants to treat them. In short, they are not protected by our laws and customs of equality. Why? Our politicians and intellectuals do not want to offend Islam by discussing the second class status of women in Islam.

When studying Islam it is necessary to study women as a separate category, because Islamic doctrine denies that men and women are equal. The duality of Islam simply makes women a separate category. The Koran has whole sections devoted to how women are treated differently from men. Many hadith describe women being treated as a special category. Islamic apologists are very proud of how Islam treats its women and says that in the West our treatment of women is terrible, that they are not protected and honored, whereas In Islam women are protected and honored.

Let's examine the doctrine that underlies the different ways women are actually treated in Islam. Islam is a rational system of politics and culture. It always has a doctrinal reason for everything it does and this is one of the things that makes studying Islam easy. If Muslims do it, there is always a reason. There is very little creativity inside of Islam. It doesn't need to be creative, because Islam has perfect doctrine which is universal and final. Its doctrine about women is perfect, therefore it doesn't need to innovate in any way. Islam even claims that it is the world's first feminist movement: that after Islam came women had more rights than before.

Let's examine the subject of the beatings of women, which is covered by Islamic doctrine. Islam means submission in all things to what Allah has revealed through Mohammed. The Koran clearly says that if a woman does not obey her husband, that is, does not submit to what he wishes, she can be beaten. Let's see how this plays out in a contemporary example. A Palestinian woman sued in a sharia court to obtain a judgment that her husband would only beat her once a week. She said that currently he beat her every day and that that was excessive. So she sued in sharia court to have them direct her husband to only beat her once a week.

The Pakistan Institute of Medical Science reported, in a scientific survey of Pakistani women, that about 90% of them said that they had been beaten by their husbands. In the country of Chad, in Africa, the national government tried to outlaw wife beatings, but Islam is quite strong in Chad. The imams and other Islamic leaders protested, saying that anti-wife beating laws were against Sharia law, and so the bill was defeated.

Some argue cynically, but practically, that since Islamic women are beaten from an early age, by the time they are married they are used to this treatment and it does not seem to bother them. This business of beating wives is thoroughly established in Islam. It is not some sort of aberration. We've already mentioned that the Koran says that the beating of a wife is permitted. Then it goes on to say that if the woman submits she should be given food, clothing, and shelter, so those are also part of a woman's rights.

Mohammed left behind a great deal of information about the beating of women. According to one hadith (tradition), Mohammed himself would hit his favorite wife, Aisha, and we know that he stood by without comment when her father struck Aisha in his presence. But then again, Mohammed also stood by without saying a word when his cousin Ali beat Aisha's black female slave. Ali was Mohammed's cousin, and also his son-in-law and the fourth man to become caliph (supreme leader) after Mohammed's death.

There's a famous hadith where a woman comes to Mohammed with a complaint about her husband. The hadith says that there was a bruise on her face which was green in color. Mohammed addressed the issue that she brought up, but he made no remark about the bruise on her face. Actually, at another time he left a hadith which said that when you hit women, do not strike them in the face. He also left behind one other piece of information on the beating of women. He said that they should be beaten lightly. This invites questions. What does it mean to beat lightly? Does it mean to use a small stick? And to use a stick, can you raise the stick above the head as you strike down at the woman? The Sunna doesn't describe this, it merely says that they are to be beaten lightly.

Islam's built-in dualities mean that Islam always has two contradictory positions. So if there is a statement that says that it is proper to beat a woman, then somewhere else there will be a contradictory statement. So, in another hadith, Mohammed said: "do not strike Allah's handmaidens." That is, don't hit women. However, there are only one or two of these statements and there are many which describe how women should be subjugated. Of course, in Islam hitting a woman is not considered abuse because hitting a woman is allowed and not forbidden. Remember, in Islam there is no "right" and "wrong" per se, but only allowed and forbidden. Beating one's wife, or another woman in one's family, is allowed and not forbidden. If the woman has been "properly" trained, she will not object to these beatings. Since Mohammed established very firmly that striking women was within the bounds of Islam, Sharia incorporates this practice into the formal structure of Islamic law. So there are rules laid out about the permitted steps by which a man makes the woman submit, with the final step being beating.

Now let's look at another way that women are treated inside of Islam. In 2002, researchers in refugee camps in Afghanistan and Pakistan found that half the girls were married by age 13. In an Afghan refugee camp more than two out of three second grade girls were either already married or engaged! Virtually all the girls who were beyond second grade were already married. One ten-year-old was engaged to a man of 60. Fifty-seven percent of Afghan girls under the age of 16 and many as young as nine are in arranged marriages. This is pure Sunna, the way of Mohammed. How do we know this? When Mohammed was in his mid-fifties, he was engaged to Aisha, a child of six. Then, when she was nine years old, he consummated the marriage. So, when the 60-year-old Pakistani Muslim is engaged to the 10-year-old it is Sunna, it is the way of Mohammed.

Now we come to a treatment of Islamic women which is not strictly Islamic doctrine, and that is "honor killings." An honor killing is when a man kills a woman because she has violated his honor. A Muslim male must control the sexuality of the females in his household or he is dishonored. It is one of his chief concerns. In Dallas, Texas two Muslim sisters were found shot to death in the back of their father's taxicab. A friend who knew them said the father was very strict about the girl's relationships with boys, their talking with boys, as well as the type of clothing the daughters wore. The sisters dressed in Western clothes and listened to popular music. The father was quite angry that his daughters were not acting like proper Muslim women.

Islamic doctrine does not explicitly authorize killing the woman who does not obey, "only" beating her. However, since a woman must be subjugated and she can be beaten, it's not too far to take the final step. But if the issue is an issue of Islam, for example, a daughter who attends a Christian church without permission, then killing her is Sunna.[3] In the story of the Battle of Bader a son is remorseful about having killed his father, who was a kafir, but in the end he realizes that since his father was a kafir, even though he was a cultured man, it was better that he was dead. So it is Sunna for one family member to kill another to advance Islam.

The Koran does specify certain rights women have. Among them are these: that they are to receive half the amount of inheritance of a male, and that in a court of law it takes the testimony of two women to equal the testimony of one man. So, if a woman testifies against a man and he denies the accusation, then the testimony has no weight at all. In Islamic court this makes cases of rape almost impossible to prove. Muslims will say: "Oh no, no, no! Islam teaches the equality of women!" Bill Warner has helpfully subjected this claim to statistical analysis (Lessons on Political Islam Level 2, "Women" p. 42). Of the 12,066 words in the Koran speaking about women, 5.3% speak highly of them, always in the context of their being mothers. 23% of the words assign equal status to women, but always in the context of Judgment Day. That's when women are equal. Then every person will be called upon to account for what they did and said in life, and in this matter men and women are to be treated equally, but there's a built-in discrepancy. It is true that the Koran says that women are to be treated equally on Judgment Day. They are to be judged on what they did in this life, and what they're supposed to do in this life is to obey the men, to submit to them, therefore, their "equality" on Judgment Day means that they will be judged on how well they submitted to men.

71% of the Koran's words about women assigns them a lower status than men. Mohammed commented that he had seen Hell and the great majority of its inhabitants were women. Why were they there? They had not fully appreciated their husbands. In the same hadith, he made the remark that women were spiritually inferior to men and that women were not as intelligent as men. Part of a woman's "rights" inside of Islam is that she's not as intelligent and she has a much better chance of going to hell. But even if she goes to Paradise, she is still in for a second-class treatment. Paradise for men is a sexual playground, but none of that seems to extend to women, so that even in Paradise, women are not rewarded like men.

This "duality" of reward in Paradise is foreshadowed by two other dualities about marriage in Islam. First, Muslim men may have up to four wives. But a Muslim woman may have only one husband. Second, it is commendable for a Muslim man to make a Christian woman his wife, because this will produce children who are raised in Islam.[4] But a Muslim woman must not, in a family which is strict about Islam, marry a Christian husband.

There's a rule about women and worship in Islam that also illustrates Islam's view of women. A man is to pray facing Mecca, and the women are to be behind him in prayer. This is the reason why women always sit in the back in the mosque.[5] Now it's interesting in the religion of Islam there are many things which can negate the power of prayer. One of those is if while you're praying a dog, a donkey or a woman walks in front of you, your prayer is nullified. So for the purposes of this tradition a woman is equal to a dog or a donkey.

Now let's take up the matter of the infamous burqa, the covering from head-to-toe which can even include the face. Some Islamic women say "Well, that is not really required." Others say that it is. Why the disagreement? Well, as you may have begun to suspect, again on this issue the Koran displays a duality of approaches. We do know this: Mohammed made all of his wives wear a veil, and that everyone in the entourage around him did so. So although there is not a universal commandment that says women should wear a burqa, we do know from the Sunna of Mohammed that his wives did and all the women around him did. This is a powerful influence with regards to the burqa.

In the Muslim holy city of Mecca, a girls' school caught on fire. Naturally, the girls tried to escape, but they were driven back into the burning building because they were not wearing their face covering and full-body veil. They died because it was the decision of the religious police that it was better they should die than have their faces exposed in the public.

Another aspect of Islam is polygamy. The Koran is quite clear on polygamy. A man may have one, two, three or four wives. It does not say that a woman can have one, two three, or four husbands.

There is also the matter of stoning. It can be argued that stoning is not Islamic, or it can be argued that it is Islamic. Here's a situation in Tehran, Iran which calls itself an Islamic republic. In 2008, two sisters, Zohre and Azar Kabiri, were convicted of adultery. They were sentenced to be stoned to death. Adultery is a crime punishable by death in Islam. In this case they first were convicted of having "illegal relations" and they were given 99 lashes each. They were brought back into court and the same evidence was used to try them for adultery, whereupon they were sentenced to be stoned to death. The evidence? It was a videotape where the two sisters were caught talking to some men without adult family members with them.

The Sharia rule about stoning is a good illustration of how detailed Sharia law can be. Sharia law says that the stones should be small enough so they do not kill immediately, but big enough so that when enough of them are thrown, they will kill the victim. Death by stoning is meant to be a torturous death that the entire community participates in.

We have just examined Islam's view of women. We must now talk about our society's response to this, which up until now has been shameful. In this country, starting in the 1960s, we had a political movement called feminism which said women should be fully equal to men before the law. There have been aspects of feminism which many Christians did not like, but it is only fair to say that politically, a great many *de facto* ways women were discriminated against were clarified. A great deal of effort has been expended to make sure women are fully equal with men before the law. But where women in Islam are concerned all of us kafirs, including "feminist" kafir women, have been shamefully silent. Consider our universities, most of which now have Women's Studies programs. Universities should be a place where issues are discussed and described but no Women's Studies departments teach anything about Sharia law for women in Islam. Outside the university, in Europe social workers do not report beatings inside Islamic families. The whole system has turned a blind eye to this.

What's happening in Europe and is starting to happen in America is this: Muslim civil rights organizations maintain that Muslims should not fall under any aspect of family law in the West because our family law is based on ignorance of Allah's law. Therefore, there should be two sets of laws, one for kafirs and one for Muslims. In other words, Muslim "civil rights" advocates want to see the duality of Islamic ethics codified into law in Europe and in America. This would mean, for example, that if a beaten Muslim woman shows up at the emergency room, the police would not be called. If she wishes to press charges, she can only do so in an Islamic court.

What is the response of Western women to this appalling inequality? Well, they don't want to be culturally insensitive. They don't want to be seen as "racist" or "Islamophobic." So if this culture of Islam wants to beat its women, they are unwilling to say anything. This kind of "tolerant multiculturalism" means that our universal human rights stop at Mohammed's door.

Islam has a precise doctrine of how to treat women. The Islamic treatment of women is that they are less than a man. That is bad enough, but what is worse is that we are not willing to help Islamic women, even those in Western countries where women supposedly have legal protection, for fear we will offend Islam. Once again, we take it for granted in America that it is ethical and moral for women to have the same rights under the law as men. But this attempt to ensure equal rights for women is only something that exists where Christianity has had a significant influence on the culture, whether directly or indirectly. It is not found in Islamic countries, because it is contrary to the Koran, the Sunna of Mohammed, and Sharia law.

QUESTIONS:

1. This chapter attempts to show that ethics in Islam and in Christianity are quite different. How would you use what you learned in this chapter to respond to a non-Muslim who asserts, based on Muslims he or she knows, that Muslims are moral people?

2. Find at least two Bible verses that help explain why the push for equal civil rights for women arose in countries influenced by Christianity and nowhere else.

Endnotes:

1   Adapted in part from Bill Warner's *Thirteen Lessons on Political Islam* Number 10 "'Ethics." May be downloaded from the Internet in its entirety at http://www.politicalislam.com/blog/category/thirteen-talks-on-political-islam/

2   Adapted in part from Bill Warner's *Thirteen Lessons on Political Islam* Number 8 "'Women." May be downloaded from the Internet in its entirety at http://www.politicalislam.com/blog/category/thirteen-talks-on-political-islam/

3   A recent example of this is the true story of Rifka Bary, a teenaged Muslim girl in Ohio who became a believer in Christ. You can see a video interview of Rifka, or read a transcript of the interview, by going to http://atlasshrugs2000.typepad.com/atlas_shrugs/2009/08/rifqa-bary-i-want-to-be-free.html

4   See, for example Married to Mohammed, by W.L. Cati Creation House Press 2001.

5   The Canadian newspaper *The Toronto Star* ran an article in its Education section on Sunday July 8, 2011 entitled "Board Runs Afoul of Education Act with Prayer Services" about the Friday Muslim prayers held during school hours in a Toronto public school to "accommodate" Muslim students. The article is accompanied by a photograph showing the girls sitting behind the boys. Sitting behind the girls are other girls, girls who are not permitted to participate in prayer because they are having their monthly menstrual period. You can view the article and the photograph at http://www.parentcentral.ca/parent/education/article/1022385--board-runs-afoul-of-education-act-with-prayer-services.

Chapter 6
Islam's Road to Triumph

Islamic Triumph by Submission & Ethical Duality

Mohammed is one of the towering figures of world history. His 1400-year impact is all the more remarkable when one realizes that up until the Hijra in AD 622 he had been successful as a businessman but not as a religious leader. For the first 13 years since his revelations began he had preached in Mecca and only gained about 150 converts. But in the last 10 years of his life he found the keys to success. His success would produce more political and military triumphs and more tears than any other single leader in history.

Here are the principles which were, and continue to be, the key to Islam's success whenever and wherever it is successful.

Jihad (literally: "striving")

Islam is to be advanced by any and every means necessary. Participating in advancing Islam by jihad of one kind or another, whether by pen or pocketbook or sword, is required of every Muslim.

Submission

"Islam" means submission. The one who submits is a "Muslim." The very term "submission" means "no compromise." Islam cannot permanently accept some nice middle ground that will allow everyone to get along, nor some secular state with all religions having equal rights and equal status. Such an arrangement can be accepted for a time to gain a strategic advantage, but it can never be a final solution because Allah has decreed that all must submit to the revelation brought by Mohammed. All of the "Dar al Harb" (the House of War) must be brought into submission to the "Dar al Islam," (the House of Submission). This means that all kafirs must either become Muslims, Dhimmis, or slaves.

Duality

We have looked at the dualistic nature of Islamic ethics. Submission is not enough to explain the success of Islam. Its most powerful principle is duality. Duality is the second major principle of Islam. We see duality in how the Koran and Mohammed's life are divided. First comes Mecca where people are permitted not to believe Mohammed, and are merely threatened with hellfire. Then comes Medina. Medina is where Jihad begins. Mohammed in Medina taught that you must submit in this life or Islam has the option of harming you. The two positions contradict each other, but both of them are held simultaneously as true.

This duality helps explain Islam's overwhelming success. Islam has two faces that it presents to the world, the face of Mecca and the face of Medina. Medina is the political and violent face. Mecca is the nice face. This lets the Koran of Mecca be used as a shield, as Teflon coating. It's the public face of Islam. Mecca is what Muslim apologists always talk about when they talk about Islam to kafirs. This duality, this subtlety, is what makes Islam so powerful because someone can't easily condemn Islam as being violent. Most Muslims are not violent at all. They are living "Mecca" Islam, practicing the "religious" side of Islam and following the Five Pillars, so therefore the charge doesn't stick.

Duality shows up when Muslims say that anything that is based upon the Koran of Medina is not the real Islam--Osama bin Laden, 9/11, al Qaeda--oh that's not the real Islam. But the duality within Islam means that two contradictory things are both true. The Muslim friend, the nice Muslim at work, is only one face of Islam. The real Islam actually includes both the Muslim friend and Osama bin Laden. The real Islam includes the Koran of Mecca (religious) and the Koran of Medina (political). In our courts of law if you take an oath as a witness, you swear: I will tell the whole truth and nothing but the truth. The "nothing but the truth" prohibits lies. But "the whole truth" prohibits something that's equally a lie, a half truth. The whole truth of Islam includes the half-truth of Mecca and the other half-truth of Medina.

The religious Koran of Mecca shields the harsh Medina Koran from public criticism. It's the Medina version that's always denied in public, but inside Islam it is known that because of the doctrine of abrogation discussed in Chapter 2 Medina outranks Mecca. Medina over Mecca is what explains another phenomenon in Islam. When something dreadful happens such as the 9/11 destruction of the World Trade Towers, the London bombings, or the Mohammed cartoon riots, Muslim spokespeople then say, "Oh, that is not the real Islam". But notice that there is never any public protest by Muslims against what has happened. There is denial, "This is not Islam," but no outrage. Why is there no protest against the violent jihadists? Because the non-violent Muslims are outranked. The Medinan Koran that celebrates war and political power abrogates the Islam of the Meccan Koran, and therefore is higher and more powerful. In the movie *The Wizard of Oz*, when Dorothy and her friends see there's a little man behind the curtain and a voice says "Oh no, no, do not look at the man behind the curtain," that is the way the duality of Mecca and Medina works. Mecca says "Oh no, do not look at the Medinan Koran behind the curtain." We kafirs are not as wise as Dorothy and Toto, so we do as we're told. We look the other way and are fooled.

We need to see the entire truth of Islam, the whole truth, not the half-truth. That's why understanding the principle of duality is an absolute necessity. If you do not understand the principle of duality you will always be fooled, lulled to sleep by the Koran of Mecca.

Let's take a current example of how duality works to shield Islam from criticism. There is a retired military man who is a devout Christian, with some Muslim friends. They pointed out to him the verses in the Koran of Mecca that sounded very good to him and they said, "This is Islam." So this Christian gentleman says, "This is very good. This is like Christianity. I like this. And besides, the Muslims are such moral people, they don't drink, their women are very modest, they don't gamble. This must be the real truth of Islam." And so he appears in public as an advocate for Islam, proclaiming that Christianity and Islam are perfectly compatible. Because of duality he does not understand that there is another truth, the truth of Medina. Because his logic is a Western logic it works like this: Jihad is contrary to the peace of Islam, so Jihad must be false; I believe in the truth of the peace of Mecca. The duality of Islam has fooled him.

But duality is present throughout the language of Islam. It uses the same words we do but with different, sometimes opposite, meanings. Take for example the word peace, *Salaam*. That sounds nice, but when you understand what Islam means by peace it's not nice at all. Peace in Islam comes only after you have submitted to Islam. That submission can be brought about by jihad. So here we have again the Koran of Mecca providing cover for the Koran of Medina. That is, our common understanding of the word "peace" hides the fact that violent jihad can be used to achieve Islamic peace.

Another example of duality is the area of women's rights. Muslims are very quick to use the phrase "women's rights" and say that Islam grants women rights. And this is true in a way, but the "rights" which Muslim women have are not the same as the rights of a Muslim man. "Women's rights" in Islam include the right to be beaten, the right to inherit half as much as a man, and the right to have their testimony worth half that of a man in court. It includes the "right" to clothing and shelter provided she pleases her husband. This duality allows a Muslim to look straight at a problem and not see the other half.

After 9/11 Muslims protested, "Oh we are the religion of peace." Because Islam maintains strict ethical duality, Muslims can say this with complete sincerity. They can think of "Islam is the religion of peace" as being absolutely true, even though they know that jihad is one of the main teachings of Islam and required of all Muslims. Duality allows a Muslim to have a totally compartmentalized mind in which the Koran of Medina never interferes with the Koran of Mecca. But deep within all the political doctrines of Islam are duality and the *kafir*. Jihad demands complete submission from the kafir and duality treats the kafir as a completely separate social and political class. Islam allows its women to be beaten to bring them into submission, but never for women to beat men. Submission comes through Duality. A separate set of rules for women. A separate set of rules for kafirs. The separate categories of kafir and women must submit.

Let's return for a moment to the issues of slavery and dhimmitude to illustrate how the principles of submission and duality work themselves out. We've already gone over in some detail Islamic slavery and its fundamental principles. Submission and duality completely explain the whole process of slavery. Who submits more than a slave? Who is so separate and apart from us? Slaves fall under a separate moral code. So submission and duality explain why slavery is completely acceptable in Islam. Or take the dhimmi and dhimmitude. Again we have the duality of a separate social and political class with its own rules. The dhimmi exists within an Islamic political system in which he is forced to submit and denied equal legal rights.

Finally there is the grand duality of all Islam — Mecca and Medina. Mecca must submit to Medina. The duality here is two separate Korans that contradict each other, but both of them completely true. We see submission and duality in Islam's ethics, with one set of rules for the believer and another set for the kafir. Islamic politics are dualistic. Everything is either in the House of Islam or the House of War. Mohammed, of course, is the chief dualist. His entire life divided into the preacher who did not do so well, and the successful jihadist -politician. Islam says it worships one, and only one, god, but that god, Allah, is the god of duality and the god of submission whom everyone is to fear. The Koran says over 300 times that we are to fear Allah.

"The fear of the Lord" is certainly a Biblical concept. Yahweh, the LORD God of the Bible, is not a fuzzy teddybear in the sky. But is this the dominant picture of God in the Bible? No. For example in Genesis, when Adam and Eve have just disobeyed and opened the floodgates of sin for the whole human race, God comes and finds them in the Garden and speaks with them (Genesis 3:8). He deals temporarily with their fallenness by providing garments of animal skins and He declares their ultimate victory over the serpent who has deceived them. If there was ever a time when people should have been afraid to be near God, it was then. Adam and Even knew this, so they hid. But God as revealed in the Bible seeks them out and talks with them. It is the same when God comes to us as Jesus. "I am found by those who sought me not" (Romans 10:20). "He is kind to the ungrateful and the evil" (Luke 6:35). "For the Son of Man came to seek and to save the lost" (Luke 19:10). In the book of Hebrews we find this: "Since therefore the children share in flesh and blood, he himself likewise partook of the same things, that through death he might destroy the one who has the power of death, that is, the devil, and deliver all those who through fear of death were subject to lifelong slavery. For surely it is not angels that he helps, but he helps the offspring of Abraham" (Hebrews 2:14-16). **In the Bible, part of the purpose of God, and even the purpose of "the fear of the Lord," is to deliver us from the bondage of the fear of death. In "Medina" Islam, the threat of death is used to produce fear and place people in bondage to Allah. There could scarcely be a starker contrast.**

Sharia[1]

Islam is a political system, a culture and a religion. The political system has a legal code called Sharia law. When most people think about Islam and possible danger to our civilization, they think of jihad. But there is something that is far more dangerous than jihad, and that is Sharia law, Islamic law. Sharia is not law in the same sense that we think of it. Sharia not only covers the normal legal things such as contracts, wills, criminal law, and how people are to be punished, but it also includes rules on how to run a family, have sex, worship, pray, say hello and other ideas that we would call religious and cultural. It even covers proper behavior in the bathroom[2]. This is because Sharia law is based upon the Koran and the Sunna. The Sunna, as we've already seen, is found in the Sira (Mohammed's biography) and the Hadith (his Traditions). Sharia law is a compilation of the directives found in the Sunna and the Koran.

Sharia law is an attempt to conform everything in a society to the society that existed in Arabia in the days of Mohammed. Sharia law can be seen as a "paper Mohammed" devoted to forcing every person to be like a Muslim Arab of Medina in 632 AD. Therefore, it goes into all the details of human life that Mohammed dictated and includes the regulation of sex, food, worship, travel and all legal details. Since Mohammed set rules for the smallest detail of life, so does Sharia.

Why is Sharia more dangerous than jihad? What most people mean by jihad is the jihad of the sword, violence. We can use police and military to protect ourselves against violence, but there is a soft jihad that comes from money, the pen and the tongue. The purpose of this "soft" jihad is to introduce Sharia law into our society and then to increase its influence. Muslims usually are in favor of this because only under Sharia law can Muslims practice pure Islam. Even those Muslims who have not lived under strict Sharia law tend to assume that such a regime is best. Of course, once Sharia is the law of the land, it is extremely difficult to change, as the now-restive population of Iran has discovered.

Sharia dictates the form of government and its laws. Pure Islam cannot be practiced in America today because we have a Constitution. But according to Sharia law, our Constitution is ignorant man-made garbage. The work that Jefferson, Adams, Benjamin Franklin and all of the other founding fathers produced is an offense to Islam. The Declaration of Independence and the Constitution are pure ignorance because they violate Sharia law and Islam. Why is it offensive? Because Benjamin Franklin and all the other people who put together our Constitution had no knowledge of any kind that mattered. How could they? According to Islam and Sharia law the only knowledge that matters comes from the Koran and the Sunna. There's nothing relevant to human beings outside of those three books — Koran, Sira, Hadith. This is what Allah has revealed, and all other merely human knowledge must submit. And therefore only laws that are based upon Koran, Sira and Hadith can be valid because man-made laws, our Constitution, all of our legal theory are nothing. They're all a part of *Jahiliya*, which means ignorance.

Our legal system is based upon two principles: the Golden Rule and critical thought. The Golden Rule is a unitary ethical system, that is, all people are to be treated the same. When we say "do unto others as you would have them do unto you," we mean ALL others, without regard to sex, race, or age. It is unitary because there is one rule, one basis of ethics. Islam is based instead on dualistic ethics because there is one set of rules for Muslims and another set of rules for kafirs. In the same way there is one set of laws for men and another set of laws for women.

Islam is not based upon critical thought, but authoritative thought. Truth is found by looking it up in the only authoritative texts: the Koran, Sira and Hadith. This means that Sharia cannot change, since the foundational texts cannot change. Sharia does not adapt. Muslims adapt to Sharia and therefore we kafirs must adapt to Sharia. Islam sneers at our Constitution because it violates all of Sharia law. Therefore as Islam comes to America, Sharia law must be triumphant.

Let's take some of our freedoms and see how they violate Islamic law. Pretend that you just woke up this morning and it is a Sharia world. What is changed? Suddenly, if you say that Mohammed made his living by taking other people's money, you go to jail. There is no freedom of speech in Islam. To contradict Islam violates Sharia law. This is because Mohammed would not tolerate being told he was wrong. When he conquered Mecca, after he prayed, he issued death warrants against those intellectuals and artists who had disagreed with him. Since Sharia is a paper Mohammed, it dictates death to those who disagree with Mohammed.

Freedom of the press is like freedom of speech. Sharia law must control the media and all artistic expression. We saw this in the Danish

Mohammed cartoons. The cartoons made fun of Islamic violence. When Muslims saw them, they turned violent and burned cities and killed people. Their response proved that the cartoonists had a valid point. But the violent response induced fear and all of the kafir newspapers submitted to Islam, practiced dhimmitude, and did not publish the cartoons. They abandoned freedom of the press. Sharia law prevailed over our Constitution. Sharia law forbids any and all artistic expression that is offensive to Islam. This means that movies, TV, the net and all art must conform to Islam in a Sharia world.

Equality of the sexes is part of our laws, but Sharia is very clear that women and men are treated differently under the law. Under Sharia, women must submit to men.

> Sura 4:34 *Allah has made men superior to women because men spend their wealth to support them. Therefore, virtuous women are obedient, and they are to guard their unseen parts as Allah has guarded them. As for rebellious women, admonish them first, and then send them to a separate bed, and then beat them.*

So the Koran says that women can be beaten. Mohammed struck his wife, and said that no one should ever ask a man why he beats his wife. Sharia even lays out exactly how a wife is beaten, what precedes the beating, and where and how she is to be struck. The submission of women does not stop with beating. In Sharia law, women's testimony in court is half that of a man's testimony. Women receive half as much as a man in an inheritance. Men have full right of divorce, but not women. The Sharia goes on and on about how to subjugate women. Women are completely subjugated inside of Sharia law. So much for all cultures being equal. Why should we tolerate any part of Sharia's subjugation of women?

In America, all categories of people can carry weapons, but under Sharia law, kafirs are forbidden to carry weapons; only Muslims may be armed. This illustrates both dualism and submission. Dualism separates kafir from Muslim. Submission means that the kafir must be in a weaker position.

Under Sharia law an apostate, one who leaves Islam, can be killed. Apostasy is the worst crime in Sharia. There is no freedom of religion. Under Sharia law, "freedom of religion" means that no one can proselytize Muslims, but Muslims can proselytize everybody. The principle of duality and submission is very clear here. In every case under Sharia there is duality and submission. Duality, because there are always two sets of laws, and submission, because the separated class, whether kafirs, women, dhimmis, slaves, or apostates must submit to Islam.

Our freedoms will have to go because they are offensive to Allah. Mohammed never allowed freedom of thought, freedom of speech, freedom of religion or freedom of the press and so Sharia does not allow those freedoms.

Our Constitution, the Declaration of Independence and Bill of Rights are the result of critical thinking based upon Biblical concepts of human nature and the Golden Rule. Both these principles and critical thinking are foreign to Sharia law. Sharia law is based upon one principle authority: the Trilogy of Koran, Sira and Hadith. The only true form of government and laws is Sharia, which means all of our civilization is jahiliyah, ignorance.

Here is how Sharia works its way into non-Islamic cultures. Muslims say: our Sharia is so precious to us; our laws are so beautiful to us that we want to be governed by our laws. Now of course, here in your country we are to follow your laws. But in matters of family, because family in Islam is very special, only the laws of Allah should rule our families. So let us use our religion and govern our own families. This includes matters such as wills, estates, divorce, domestic abuse, and adoption. All of these things are nothing to you because we are separate from you. It's just a matter of how we run our own families.

Now this seems innocent enough to politicians or to "intellectuals" who know nothing of Islam. It is especially welcome in the modern West because the multicultural idea is that all cultures are equally valid, so "of course" Muslims must be allowed to follow their own culture. But in the process of welcoming sharia, we are submitting to it, because "making space" for Sharia is allowing Islam to do things its own way. Does it matter to us how a Muslim writes a will? Hmm, seems like a small thing, nothing to worry about. Or is it really? Think about property ownership whose transfer is no longer subject to the scrutiny of American courts. In England there are already many Sharia courts set up to rule over Muslims. England has effectively entered into two parallel systems of law, a legal dualism which means it has given up its sovereignty.

Sharia is the longest wedge in the world and the thin end of it is firmly in place in England, but it is also already in place in America. In America in cities where Muslims congregate to create their own societies, Sharia law is already in place. In certain areas of America today, a Muslim woman does not call the police if she is beaten, because the Muslim community will turn against her. A Muslim husband can beat his wife under Sharia law. The Islamic community enforces Sharia in the areas it controls. This is the practical implementation of Sharia law in America, and it is gaining traction in American courts. Consider the following article, published at http://shariahinamericancourts.com.

New Study Finds Shariah Law Involved in Court Cases in 23 States

Washington, DC, May 17, 2011 — The Center for Security Policy today released an in-depth study-- *Shariah Law and American State Courts: An Assessment of State Appellate Court Cases*. The study evaluates 50 appellate court cases from 23 states that involve conflicts between Shariah (Islamic law) and American state law. The analysis finds that Shariah has been applied or formally recognized in state court decisions, in conflict with the Constitution and state public policy.

Some commentators have tried to minimize this problem, claiming, as an editorial in yesterday's *Los Angeles Times* put it that, "...There is scant evidence that American judges are resolving cases on the basis of shariah." To the contrary, our study identified 50 significant cases just from the small sample of appellate court published cases.

Others have asserted with certainty that state court judges will always reject any foreign law, including Shariah law, when it conflicts with the Constitution or state public policy. The Center's analysis, however, found 15 trial court cases, and 12 appellate court cases, where Shariah was found to be applicable in these particular cases.

The facts are the facts: some judges are making decisions deferring to Shariah law even when those decisions conflict with constitutional protections.

On releasing the study, the Center for Security Policy's President, Frank J. Gaffney, Jr., observed:

> "These cases are the stories of Muslim American families, mostly Muslim women and children, who were asking American courts to preserve their rights to equal protection and due process. These families came to America for freedom from the discriminatory and cruel laws of Shariah. When our courts then apply Shariah law in the lives of these families, and deny them equal protection, they are betraying the principles on which America was founded."

The implementation of Sharia within the American judicial system is the most dangerous form of jihad now being practiced against America and Western Europe, far more society-altering in the long run than acts of terror.

The Tears of Jihad[3]

The Tears of Jihad refers to the deaths of 270 million people over a 1400 year period. They were all killed for the same reason. They did not believe that Mohammed was the prophet of Allah.

Mohammed was the most successful military and political leader who ever lived, because he not only succeeded at conquering during his lifetime, but beyond, for 1400 years. We have other examples in history of men who became all-powerful in their lifetime. We can measure to some degree how

HELPING CHRISTIANS UNDERSTAND *Islam*

powerful they were by how many people they caused to die. The person who we usually think of as having killed the most people was Mao Tse-Tung. As far as we can tell, through starvation, persecution and outright executions, Mao Tse-Tung was responsible for the death of 77 million people.

Now compare this to Mohammed, who through his principle of jihad and its aggressive politics has caused the death of at least 270 million people over 1400 years. Mao killed 77 million just within his lifetime. But the total of those that Mao killed is far fewer than those who have been and are being killed in imitation of Mohammed. Since 9/11, over 58,000 worldwide have been killed in the name of Mohammed, and that number increases almost daily. 58,000 dead is equivalent to all the Americans killed in the Vietnam War. When we think of a powerful political leader we may think of Napoleon, or of Alexander the Great or Caesar. They were great generals and powerful politicians, but they don't hold a candle to Mohammed, because no one today kills for Napoleon's cause. No one today kills for Caesar. But today as you are reading these words, it is undoubtedly true that somewhere in the world people are being destroyed by other people who are zealously following the perfect example of Mohammed.

After Mohammed died, Abu Bakr was elected Caliph, Supreme Ruler of all Islam. He, like every subsequent Caliph, was responsible for both spiritual guidance and political guidance, because the spiritual and the political are not separated in Islam. The Caliph was a combination of pope and emperor. Abu Bakr spent his three years in office making sure that Muslim Arabs did not leave Islam. Apostasy which is not repented from calls for the death penalty in Islam. Umar was the next Caliph after Abu Bakr died. Umar was the Caliph, you'll remember, who "standardized" the text of the Koran. When it came to killing, he picked up where Mohammed left off. Mohammed's last efforts were all directed toward attacking the Christians north of Arabia. They were kafirs. They had not submitted to Islam. So attacking Christians was the focus of Umar's caliphate.

At this time, the Middle East was not remotely like what we think of now. It was basically a Greek culture. What had happened was that the Greeks were sailors and businessmen and so the Greek culture, what historians call "Hellenistic culture" (from "Hellas" meaning "Greece"), spread all around the rim of the Mediterranean, including Syria and Northern Egypt. North Africa was a Greek culture. All of Anatolia (what is now Turkey) was Greek. It was a highly sophisticated culture but it had overwhelming problems by the 700s: age, degeneracy and decay.

The Greeks had been at war with the Persians for a long time. This continual war left both the Persians and the Greeks weak, so the 900 year rule of Greek culture in the Mediterranean was coming to an end. The Greeks were also very divided along religious lines. Christianity had several variations and the Greeks in Constantinople had a different kind of Christianity than was held in Jerusalem, Syria and Egypt. These divisions were strong enough to cause ill will. So it was a divided Hellenistic world that Umar invaded and conquered. The conquest went so fast that Umar was not really able to govern what he had conquered, but on the other hand he now had enormous wealth because Syria fell, Persia fell, and Iraq, Egypt, and North Africa all fell to Islam. In thirty years time all of Greek culture except what was in Anatolia (what is now Turkey) and Greece itself was destroyed. An entire new world order came about.

At first the conquered Christians were left pretty much to govern themselves and only send taxes to Medina. This interim is sometimes cited as evidence for the "mildness" of Islamic conquest. But after the consolidation of the empire under Uthman, the next Caliph, things began to change. Islam was no longer conquering more territory, instead it was consolidating. The age of the dhimmi had arrived. Being a dhimmi involved paying heavy taxes, but it also meant becoming a second class citizen in your own home country. In Egypt, for instance, the Coptic culture was especially despised. The Copts, the descendants of the Egypt of the Pharaohs, had become Christians. The Coptic language was thousands of years old, but if as a Christian you spoke the Coptic language in front of your new Arab masters, your tongue was cut out. That was the life of the dhimmi. North Africa became Islamic. 600 years of Christianity disappeared. The culture of the Greeks and the Romans, the Europeans, was annihilated. Then the pressure started up against Greek Anatolia.

Everywhere the Muslims looked, they saw Christians who were wealthy, educated and very sophisticated. The Arabs were none of these things. They just wanted to crush the Christian kafirs, so the 900-year-old world of the Middle East completely changed. And notice something: it has not changed in the last 1400 years except to become even more Islamic.

The Christians had no idea what hit them. They could not even properly identify their attackers. They never called the invaders Muslims, instead they called them Arabs or Saracens. In Spain they were called "Moors." Here is a quote written by Christians attacked at that time.

> "The sword of the Saracen, beastly and demonic savages. Evil God-hating Saracens destroyed crops, burned cities and drove the survivors before them."

The poor Christians at that time did not understand that their enemy was Islam. Today we face the same kind of attacks from the same enemy. Our enemy is not "terrorism." "Terrorism" is a tactic. It is one way to conduct jihad. No, our enemy is the same as the Christians of the early Medieval Mediterranean world. It is the ideology promoted by Mohammed through the Medinan Koran, the Hadith, and the Sira, the ideology named "Islam," or, in Bill Warner's helpful phrase, "political Islam."

After the Middle East was conquered, Arab Muslims looked towards Constantinople, the Byzantine Roman capital in Anatolia. This became a long term goal which took a few hundred years to accomplish. Their first step was to kill Armenians. In one town they brought together all of the Armenian leaders, took them down to the church and burned the church and it fell in on top of them. In another town in Anatolia, when a Christian came to pay the dhimmi tax, he was branded with a hot iron on the arm. If anyone was found without this brand, the arm that should have held the brand was cut off. It didn't hurt very long because the next thing cut off was his head.

There was one Greek Bishop who offered to debate the Muslims with regards to Islam and Christianity. The Muslims listened to his debate for two hours then they cut off his head. Another Bishop invited them to a debate so they too, debated for the afternoon. When the debate was over the Muslims took the bishop, cut out his tongue, hauled him out to the desert and left him to die.

Needless to say, acts like this began to teach the Christians what their place was in this new order. It was a place of the dhimmi, a semi-slave. They could still have their church buildings, those that were left. Christianity could not be seen or spoken of beyond the church or the home. For a Christian to try to convert a Muslim was a death sentence.

Christians were actually forbidden to read the Koran. This element is important because it helped to ensure ignorance about their Islamic rulers on the part of the Christians. This has had a 1,400-year effect. Christians and other kafirs like the Israelis still do not study either the history or the doctrine of Islam. This makes anyone, including a Christian, a likely candidate for dhimmitude, because dhimmitude starts with ignorance. The prevention and cure for dhimmitude is knowledge. Once a dhimmi becomes aware of the Islamic doctrine of jihad and the history of Islamic persecution of kafirs, the dhimmi's eyes are opened to all of what Islam is. The dhimmi becomes determined to remain a kafir, that is, one who does not submit to Islam.

The destruction in Anatolia continued over several hundred years. We have one accounting from a Muslim historian who proudly reports the destruction of 30,000 church buildings. Some of the nicer church buildings had a special fate reserved for them. Those sites became mosques. When it has conquered, Islam has built its mosques on top of where the best church building or temple was. This is Sunna, the way of Mohammed, because it is what Mohammed did when he conquered Mecca. He converted the pagan temple into Islam's holiest shrine.

Destroying religious art is also the way of Mohammed. As soon as Islam conquered any town, the churches were desecrated. The Christians could move back into them later if Islam decided to let them stand. Art, in particular religious art, is an affront to Islam, it is considered tantamount to idolatry. So Mohammed's first act on returning to Mecca was to pray. His next act was to destroy all the religious art, and his example has been followed everywhere Islam conquers. We see this in Egypt, for instance, where the nose of the Sphinx was knocked off. We see this along the silk route where all of the Buddhist murals in caves have had the eyes pecked out and the mouth taken out. It was Islam that invented the word "deface," because this is literally what was done to all religious art.

Over the hundreds of years it took for Islam to fully subdue Anatolia, there was an interesting side effect for those who had already been conquered elsewhere. If the Arabs lost a battle in Anatolia, then back in Egypt, for example, there would be riots of anger because the Christians had defeated the Muslims, and Christians conveniently under Muslim control would be killed. This is the same pattern that recently produced the killing of innocent Christians after the cartoons of Mohammed were published, and after the Florida pastor announced the burning of a Koran.

This persecution was what set the stage for Christians in the Middle East to cry out to their brothers in Europe, and the response of the Europeans in the Crusades was to try to help them. The history of the crusades is one of the few times where Christians tried to help other Christians in the Middle East. The Crusades began out of good intentions. Both their successes and their failures should be studied to glean what can be done to help Christians who are oppressed by Islam, and what ought, and ought not, to be done.

In the Middle East, jihad was not just against the Christians, it was against everyone. The Persian Empire at this time had already been crushed. Zoroastrianism, the religion of the Persians, was annihilated. So was the Nestorian form of Christianity which had spread in what is now Iran and Iraq, and even into western China. The Zoroastrians were so badly crushed that today historians are not really sure of the true nature of Zorastrianism because so many of its sacred texts were destroyed. Islam then moved towards Hindustan, or India. Due to jihad, what we think of as India today is about half of its original territory. But on the way to Hindustan, Islam stopped off in Afghanistan and destroyed the Buddhism that was there.

They then turned to the Hindus. The attack against the Hindus was similar to the ones against the Christians, Buddhists and Persians. When

Islam started attacking the Persians, there was a parlay, a conference before the battle, and the Persian general asked "Who are you and why are you here?" because the Persians had never really fought the Arabs. And here, in a hadith, is what the Islamic military commander told him. "Our prophet, the messenger of our Lord, has ordered us to fight you until you worship Allah alone or pay the jizyah, the dhimmi tax, and our prophet has informed us that our Lord says whoever amongst us is killed shall go to paradise and lead a life of great luxury. Whoever amongst us remains alive will become your master." This is a perfect statement of the rationale for Jihad, a rationale that has not changed, because it is based upon the words and example of Mohammed.

Similar is the statement by one of the conquering Muslim generals of India, Tamerlane. "My principle aim in coming to Hindustan has been to accomplish two goals. The first is to war with the kafirs, the enemies of Mohammed, and by this holy war, be able to claim a reward in paradise. The other is that the army of Islam may gain by plundering the wealth of the kafirs. Plunder in war is as lawful as a mother's milk to a Muslim."

You can see that the reason for invading Hindustan was exactly the reason for invading Persia and that the same reason lay behind invading Anatolia and the Middle East. It's important to realize this because many times people think that when the Muslims invaded maybe the people they invaded were just getting what was coming to them. No, their only fault was to be kafirs. The Greeks, the Persians, and the Hindus were all kafirs.

Just as the culture of the Middle East was crushed, the culture of the Hindu was crushed. Islam changed the Hindu. Before Islam the Hindus had been a proud culture. They were a leader in intellectual theory, mathematics and philosophy, and they were very wealthy. Hindustan had been an Empire for a thousand years. It had been relatively peaceful, and peaceful times allow prosperity. That was one of the things that happened in Afghanistan with the Buddhists. They were very prosperous because they had given up war. It turns out that the Buddhists show what happens when you deal with Islam on the basis of "we are peaceful people, we will do whatever you want." What happened to the peaceful Buddhists was that the pacifists were annihilated. Half of the Hindu culture still remains behind because it had a warrior caste. None of the Buddhist culture remains in Afghanistan.

Here is a typical story from the Islamic conquest of India. 20,000 Jihadists and thousands of mercenaries laid siege to a city in Hindustan. For money, a traitor in the city gave them a clue as to how they could place ladders up against one particular portion of the wall and penetrate the city. The Muslims poured into the city. For three days they did nothing but kill. They didn't even rob the bodies. The Muslim General gave the job of killing the Hindus to only his most religious men, as they would press on and not be distracted by plunder. After three days they stopped the killing and then began to rob the bodies. While the killing was going on, women and children were raped, because rape always accompanies violent jihad. Rape is another way of subduing the kafirs and forcing them to submit. In the end the Hindus were crushed. Half their territory was gone. They were sold into slavery. There are some remnants of this in the geography books. For example, there is in Afghanistan a mountain range called the Hindu Kush. Hindu Kush means the funeral pyre of the Hindu.

What we now call Pakistan, which means "Holy Land," was originally part of India. The partition of Pakistan after World War II was done so that it would become purely Islamic. This happened under British supervision. About a million Hindus were killed in the partition that led to the creation of the state of Pakistan. It was Ghandi, the secular saint, whose decisions led to these deaths. His pacifist principles were ultimately disarming to the British, and led to Indian independence, because the British were grounded in a biblical ethic. But the Islamic leaders who established Pakistan were operating under a different ethic. Ghandi, seeking to be a reconciler, said that although all of the Hindus had to leave Pakistan, none of the Muslims in India had to leave. He was trying to be kind to Muslims and accommodating to the Islamic leaders of Pakistan, but the result was a million dead Hindus, plus many more Muslims and Hindus killed in the counter-reaction riots that erupted in India itself. Today, the Muslims remaining in India are an ongoing political problem. After Indonesia, the second-largest number of Muslims in the world live in India. So both Ghandi and the peaceful Buddhists of Afghanistan show that simply giving in to Islamic political expansion does not work.

On the opposite side of India, in Bangladesh, Islamicization goes on today. In 1947 Bangladesh was still about one-third Hindu. Today it is about 10% Hindu. And the reduction of the Hindus has come at a terrible cost. Hindu women and men in Bangladesh are persecuted on a daily basis. For example, the police turn a blind eye when some Muslim throws acid in a Hindu woman's face because her face is not veiled. The police will not investigate because the police are Muslim.

The first September 11th was in 1683 when the Europeans drove the Muslims from the gates of Vienna. Some years later we had another September 11th, and here's what is significant about that. Islam never forgot that it was on September 11th it had been turned back from the gates of Vienna and the proud Turkish Army defeated. Islam never forgot, but on September 11th in America we had no idea why that date was chosen. We were clueless. In our cluelessness we see the nature of both Islam and the kafir. The kafir never remembers the history of the expansion of Islam, while Islam never forgets.

Since 9/11 more than 58,000 people around the world have died in more than 9,000 attacks, and the number increases daily. More than 87,000 have been injured in 39 countries. All of this suffering goes on around the world and we hear about only a tiny portion of it. Our press apparently does not want to report the terror of what the political agenda of Islam is producing around the world.

But we can't blame just our press, because none of our schools teach the history of the Tears of Islam. Not even the Christian schools teach the dreadful history of the destruction of 60 million Christians. No schools teach the deaths of 10 million Buddhists, 80 million Hindus and 120 million Africans.

And since we don't know this history it looks at this point as if we are doomed to repeat it. Islam continues to kill the kafir and the kafir just says "Oh well, we'll take care of that problem by pretending it is not there." The reason we won't turn our attention to it is complicated, but part of it has to do with the shame of the history, because the kafir has been defeated time and again by Islam. We absolutely refuse to admit that Islam is a culture that, as a matter of sacred duty, is devoted to the annihilation of kafir culture. This is not an "Islamophobic" kneejerk reaction. The proof is all around us. When you go to Iraq, you no longer find a Christian Iraq. When you go to Egypt, you no longer find a Christian Egypt. It is Islamic.

There's only one way to respond to this. The history of the Tears of Jihad must be taught in our kafir schools. How can it be that we are taught, correctly, about the evil history of America slavery, but nothing about the 14 million Africans enslaved and 120 million Africans killed in the name of Islam? How can we treat the history of the expansion of the empire of Islam as a glorious history but ignore the history of the suffering of the dhimmis and the death of over 270 million, especially when the Tears of Jihad continue to fall today? How can we allow our children to believe that a legal system that discriminates against women and favors one religion over all others should be allowed any standing whatsoever in a free society?

QUESTIONS:

1. What do you think you would most dislike about living under Sharia law?

2. Why do you think many Western intellectuals who think Christianity is oppressive are so willing to accommodate Islam?

Endnotes:

1   Adapted in part from Bill Warner's _Thirteen Lessons on Political Islam_ Number 13 "'Sharia." May be downloaded from the Internet in its entirety at http://www.politicalislam.com/blog/category/thirteen-talks-on-political-islam/

2   Keller, _The Reliance of the Traveler_, pp. 75-79.

3   Adapted in part from Bill Warner's _Thirteen Lessons on Political Islam_ Number 14 "'The Tears of Jihad." May be downloaded from the Internet in its entirety at http://www.politicalislam.com/blog/category/thirteen-talks-on-political-islam/

Concluding Thoughts

"**A**llah did not create man so that he could have fun. The aim of creation was for mankind to be put to the test through hardship and prayer. An Islamic regime must be serious in every field. There are no jokes in Islam. There is no humor in Islam. There is no fun in Islam. There can be no fun and joy in whatever is serious. Islam does not allow swimming in the sea and is opposed to radio and television serials. Islam, however, allows marksmanship, horseback riding and competition ..."

Ayatollah Ruhollah Khoimeini, founder of the current Islamic Republic of Iran — Quoted in Wikipedia http://en.wikipedia.org/wiki/Political_thought_and_legacy_of_Khomeini#Sternness source: Meeting in Qom "Broadcast by radio Iran from Qom on 20 August 1979," quoted in Taheri, *The Spirit of Allah* (1985) p.259)

"*the joy of the LORD is your strength*" (**Nehemiah 8:10**)

"*looking to Jesus, the founder and perfecter of our faith, who for the joy that was set before him endured the cross ...*" (**Hebrews 12:2**)

"**Q. 1. What is the chief end of man?**
A. Man's chief end is to glorify God, and to enjoy him forever."
(**Westminster Shorter Catechism**)

121

What a contrast! A condemnation of joy, and an invitation to joy! Throughout this book the attempt has been made to show how very, very different the worldviews are of Islam and Christianity. The source of authority is different. The nature of God is different. The ethical principles are different. The kind of politics and culture that either developed (Christianity) or is prescribed (Islam) is different. The eternal hope offered is different.

In addition to Islam, the other powerful cultural force that erodes Christianity in our day is post-modernist relativism. That is, the belief that all cultures and belief systems are equally good. The impossibility of this being true is proven by totalitarian belief systems, of which Islam is one. How can a culture and belief system that requires everyone to submit to it be equal to one that allows each individual to believe as he or she wishes? Someone may well believe that the totalitarian system, whether communism, fascism, or Islam, is superior, but it is impossible for it to be equal to a system that allows freedom of belief and action. One cannot embrace both. One must choose which is better for individuals and societies. In this other arena of ideas Islam may be doing Christianity and the West a favor by exposing the hollowness of post-modernist relativism.

Moreover, public law and policy must be based on some ethical standard. Most Western laws, including laws championed by those who say "don't legislate morality," are based on the ethic of the Golden Rule: do to others as you want them to do to you. But law based on a totalitarian ethic will inevitably mean "some are more equal than others." Under communism, it was Communist Party members, and especially Party leaders, who operated under one law, while another law governed everybody else. Under Islam, there is one law for Muslims, especially religious leaders, and another law for everybody else (kafirs).

Biblically-based Christianity, for all the flaws of its practitioners, and there are many flaws, has somehow in God's Providence produced a culture where each individual, at least theoretically, has value. It took a long, painful process to get here, shedding slavery and the oppression of minorities and women in the process. The current resurgence of Islam is an invitation to lose every principle of liberty the West has gained since the time of Mohammed. Or, we can refuse the invitation of Islam and issue our own invitation.

We can seize every opportunity to love Muslims, while telling them that God is love, loves them, and invites them to know Him personally.

We can seize every opportunity to tell Muslims the truth about Jesus, inviting them to read what the New Testament says about Him. It is important that Muslims learn that Christian beliefs are based on the Bible, since the Koran does commend the Christian Scriptures.

We can pray for Muslims corporately, and also, whenever they would like it, individually. Our loving Savior will act in their lives as we invite Him.

Many Muslims are described by the words of Paul, the former Saul of Tarsus, persecutor of Christians: *"I bear them witness that they have a zeal for God, but not according to knowledge. For being ignorant of the righteousness that comes from God, and seeking to establish their own, they did not submit to God's righteousness"* (**Romans 10:2-3**). What an irony! The belief system that stresses "submission" to God is seeking to establish its own righteousness, and thereby actually failing to submit to the Only One who brings the righteousness of God, namely Jesus Christ.

Now that you have the facts about Islam as a system, set them aside when interacting with Muslims. Remember that most Muslims don't read Arabic. Even those who do have usually read only portions of the Koran, and little or none of the Hadith or Sira. So you must take time in each case to learn what your Muslim friend or acquaintance knows and believes about Islam. Among those who have chosen to live in a non-Islamic society, there is often a wide variety of knowledge and belief.

Don't attack Mohammed or Islam, it will only make your Muslim friends defensive. Instead, learn truthful responses to their questions, responses that are less likely to raise red flags. For example, don't start by insisting that Jesus is the Son of God. Remember, for Muslims, they think when we say this we mean that God had sex with Mary! If and when the subject comes up, a helpful way to respond is to ask: "Can God can do anything He wants to?" Yes, of course He can, and Muslims believe this! So then explain that when Christians call Jesus "the Son of God," they mean that God chose to visit earth as a man, the man Jesus of Nazareth, the Christ (Messiah), which means the One Anointed by the Holy Spirit. You may want to show them a place like the Gospel of Mark 1:9-11 where the Spirit comes upon Jesus and immediately the voice of God from heaven says "You are my beloved Son." As the Holy Spirit opens their hearts, they will embrace more and more of the truth about who Jesus is. Their heart may well believe before their mind is fully convinced.

Much more helpful information in trying to explain Christianity to Muslims can be found at one of the resources listed at the end of this book, www.answering-islam.org. This website answers Muslims' questions in a number of different languages, so even if they don't speak English well, they can read answers in what is probably their native language, such as Arabic, Persian, Indonesian, Urdu, Turkish, and other languages.

Finally, in our responsibility as free citizens of a democratic Republic, we must do our best to explain to others why Islam as a political system is not compatible with a free society. Give political support to leaders who understand this, and who will resist allowing Sharia law to govern people who live in the United States under our Constitution. There is no conflict under our Constitution with purely "religious" Islam. Muslims can and should be free to attend mosque, wash before prayers, and practice fasting on Ramadan. But permitting multiple marriages, wife-beating, or granting special favors in schools and the workplace, favors not given to other students and workers, is to concede hard-won ground to a totalitarian system that always presses for one-way submission, not for mutual respect and cooperation. There is an analogy to the American Communist Party during the Cold War. The Communists were allowed to live without being persecuted, to speak, and to field candidates just like any other party. They were NOT allowed special privileges denied other parties. Neither should Muslims be allowed special privileges and exemptions from the law just because they are Muslims.

An honest comparison of Christianity and Islam, including God as presented in Christianity and Islam, can only cause the superiority of Christ to shine. There's no need to attack Islam when speaking with Muslims. Honest questions to provoke thoughtful discussion can be good, but in every case, love Muslims and lift up Christ.

Jesus loves Muslims with an everlasting love. He loves them right now, but they are ignorant of it. Fear of family and community can choke out any impulse they have to seek Him. Islam, which began in opposition to idols, puts a huge idol in the path of any Muslim seeking to know the living God, an idol called "the opinion of the Muslim community." We are called as followers of Jesus to love them anyway, even those who right now are refusing to come to Him. They are lost and don't know it. They are children blundering in the dark and the wolf is at hand. They don't know how to find God. So we are called to snatch them from the darkness and the fire of destruction (Jude 23). The price of the Cross was paid for them, too! So wherever we find them ready to hear, we must welcome them in.

We live in a time like our Lord described in the banquet parable of Luke 14. All over the world, the Lord of the banquet is sending His servants to the remote, unreached people and by the force of love compelling many who have never heard the Gospel before to come in and dine with Him.[1] The Bride is being prepared! It is a Kingdom hour. While in the past the light has shown at times and in various places, God has granted us to live in a time when it will shine across the world, including the Muslim world. The knowledge of the glory of God will cover the earth as the water covers the sea (Habakkuk 2:14). Rejoice!

Endnotes:

1   ANM is in the privileged position of hearing many true stories of how God is doing this right now. Here is one example from North Africa. A Muslim father was deeply concerned that his son was becoming involved with a militant jihadist group, as he feared for his son's life. One night he had a dream in which his son was falling into a deep well. A man in dressed in white appeared and took his son by the hand. But something was continuing to pull the son down, and the man in white said to the father: "I cannot bring

him out unless he lets go what is in his hand." The father looked and in the son's hand was a Koran. Then the son let it go, and the man in white drew him out of the well. The father went looking for an explanation of his dream, and received it from an indigenous Christian. The father gave his life to Christ, and later, so did the son. For more stories, go to www.adnamis.org.

Appendix 1
Muslim Jihad in Christian Ethiopia
Lessons for the West

by Raymond Ibrahim
FrontPageMagazine.com
March 28, 2011 *(Reproduced by permission of the author)*

Not only does last week's jihadist rampage against Ethiopia's indigenous Christians highlight the travails Christians encounter wherever Islam has a sizable population, but it offers several insights, including some which should concern faraway, secular nations with Muslim minorities. According to Fox News:

Thousands of Christians have been forced to flee their homes in Western Ethiopia after Muslim extremists set fire to roughly 50 churches and dozens of Christian homes. At least one Christian has been killed, many more have been injured and anywhere from 3,000 to 10,000 have been displaced in the attacks that began March 2 after a Christian in the community of Asendabo was accused of desecrating the Koran.

For starters, this "medieval" attack is a reminder that countless churches have been destroyed or desecrated by jihadist terror since Islam rose to power in the Medieval era, evincing centuries of continuity. While the media may mention the more "spectacular" attacks on churches—in <u>Iraq</u>, in <u>Egypt</u>—most attacks go either <u>unreported or underreported</u>. (Some Muslim nations, such as U.S. "friend-and-ally" Saudi Arabia, nip it in the bud by outlawing churches in the first place.)

Moreover, the dubious excuse used to justify this latest barbarous outburst—"desecration of the Koran"—is a reminder of the double-standards Bibles suffer in the Islamic world, where they are routinely confiscated and burned. Indeed, even as Muslim Ethiopians were rampaging, Muslim nations hailed as being "moderate"—<u>Malaysia</u> and <u>Bangladesh</u>—also made headlines last week with their deplorable treatment of Christians and Bibles. Worse, the West helps standardize such a biased approach: the U.S. government—Obama, Hillary, and any number of other grandstanding politicians—rose up in condemnation when a virtually anonymous, small-town pastor threatened to burn the Koran, while saying nary a word about the countless Bibles daily mutilated in the Muslim world (a <u>2003 fatwa</u> that ruled the Bible suitable for use by Muslims when <u>cleaning after defecation</u> went largely unnoticed).

Such a gutless approach is not surprising considering the sort of people who advise the military, such as Lt. Cmdr. Youssef Aboul-Enein, who recommends that, if ever an American soldier desecrates a Koran, U.S. leadership must offer "unconditional apologies," and emulate the words of Maj. Gen. Jeffrey Hammond: "I come before you [Muslims] seeking your forgiveness, in the most humble manner I look in your eyes today, and say please forgive me and my soldiers," followed by abjectly kissing a new Koran (*Militant Islamist Ideology*, p. 26).

Finally, for those Western observers who live beyond the moment and have an interest in the big picture, the long run—the world bequeathed to future generations—the issue of numbers revealed by this Ethiopian anecdote should give cause to pause. The Fox News report continues:

The string of attacks comes on the heels of several reports of growing anti-Christian tension and violence around the country where Muslims make up roughly one-third of the total population but more than 90 percent of the population in certain areas, 2007 Census data shows. One of those areas is Besheno where, on November 9, all the Christians in the city woke up to find notes on their doors warning them to convert to Islam, leave the city or face death.

As Jonathan Racho, an official at International Christian Concern, said, "It's extremely disconcerting that in Ethiopia, where Christians are the majority, they are also the victims of persecution." This oddity is explained by Prime Minister Meles Zenawi's assertion that Ethiopian Islamists "have changed their tactics and they have been able to camouflage their activities through legal channels"—a strategy regularly implemented by Islamists wherever they are outnumbered, like in the U.S., prompting countermeasures such as Islamist Watch and the Legal Project.

That Muslims are an otherwise peaceable minority group in Ethiopia, but in enclaves where they represent the majority, they attack their outnumbered Christian countrymen—giving them a tweaked version of Islam's three choices to infidels—suggests that Muslim aggression and passivity are very much rooted in numbers: the more Muslims, the more potential for "assertive" behavior.

This has lessons for the West, especially Europe, which in recent years has seen an unprecedented influx of Muslim immigrants, reaching some 53 million, a number expected to "nearly double by 2015, while the non-Muslim will shrink by 3.5%," due to higher Muslim birth rates. In short, it is a matter of time before Muslims account for significant numbers in Europe—perhaps not the majority, but, as the Ethiopian example establishes, a majority is not necessary for the winds of jihad to blow.

Indeed, the story of Islam's entry into Ethiopia, one of the oldest Christian civilizations, is illustrative. Around 615, when the pagan Quraysh were persecuting Muhammad's outnumbered Muslim followers in Arabia, some fled to Ethiopia seeking sanctuary. The

Christian king, or "Negus" of Ethiopia, welcomed and protected these Muslim fugitives, ignoring Quraysh demands to return them—and thus winning Muhammad's gratefulness. Today, 14 centuries later, when Islam has carved itself a solid niche in Ethiopia, accounting for 1/3 of the population, Muslim gratefulness has turned to something else—not least a warning to Western states.

Appendix 2
Women in Osama Bin Laden's Thinking

In her Internet article <u>Was Osama a Typical Husband and Father?</u> (http://frontpagemag.com/2011/05/04/was-osama-a-typical-husband-and-father/), Phyllis Chesler writes:

"In Growing Up Bin Laden, Osama's first wife/first cousin, Najwa bin Laden, and his fourth son, Omar bin Laden, (Najwa's son too), reveal Osama's monstrous but rather typical behavior vis-a-vis women and children, including his own.

Bin Laden, the holy warrior, had four-five wives (Najwa Ghanem, Khadijah Sharif, Khairiah Sabar, Siham Sabar, and Amal Al-Sadah who replaced his annulled fifth marriage and/or his divorced wife, Khadijah Sharif). Osama fathered eleven sons and eight daughters (nineteen children), ten with Najwa alone. According to Najwa and Omar, Osama was not physically cruel to his wives. He never beat them or raised his voice to them. They were chosen for their submissiveness, passivity, and religiosity. Typically, like many Arab and Muslim men, Osama loved his mother; he may even have identified with her as a kindred outcast. His first wife, Najwa, was his mother's niece. He and Najwa lived with Osama's mother, Allia, for a long time.

To Osama, women were important as breeders and domestic servants but otherwise they did not really matter, they were not important. He spent most of his time with other men, warriors or businessmen. His first wife was fifteen years old. Osama expected a wife to "know her place." He expected his four wives to live in purdah (to observe the strictest Saudi or Afghan style face and body coverings). Despite his enormous wealth, Osama condemned his wives to very primitive living conditions, and essentially expected them to work as domestic beasts of burden. He never concerned himself with their comfort and forced them to live in austere settings with little furniture. However, his relationship to Najwa was one of mutual understanding and tenderness.

Still, according to her son and co-author, Omar, even when Najwa was suffering from a difficult pregnancy, 'she lived without air-conditioning in the hottest weather, without proper heating in the coldest weather, without modern appliances to store or cook food or wash her family's clothes, without proper food for her children, without medical care for anyone and without a way of communicating with her mother and siblings.'

Najwa never complained and maintained the "sweetest composure."

Osama the mighty warrior could or would not live for long without his women and children with him. He took them along into danger and privation. He dragged all his wives and children along with him, first to Saudi Arabia, then into exile, in Sudan, and Afghanistan where he literally demanded that they live in a cave. Najwa left Afghanistan two days before 9/11. At least one wife, probably his fifth wife Amal, stayed with him and accompanied him to Pakistan. She is the one who may have functioned as his "human shield" in his final confrontation with American Navy Seals.

What I am about to say will probably be minimized if not dismissed by serious foreign policy wonks but here goes: according to his son, Osama's final straw in deciding to wage war on America was not his ongoing feud with the Saudi royal family, but rather the presence of infidel female soldiers on Saudi and Muslim soil, brought there to protect Saudi men. Omar writes:

> "At the first sight of a capable-looking female soldier, my father became the most outspoken opponent of the royal decision to allow Western armies into the Kingdom, ranting, 'Women! Defending Saudi men!' No insult could be worse. My father became frustrated to the point of declaring that he could not longer accept the pollution he claimed hung in the air above any non-Muslim."

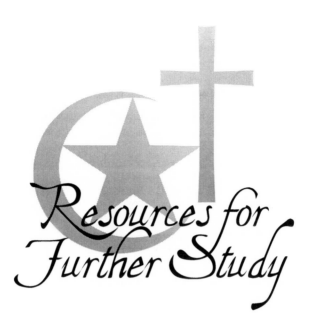

Resources for Further Study

The Decline of Eastern Christianity Under Islam by Bat Ye'or

The Politically Incorrect Guide to Islam (and the Crusades) by Robert Spencer

The Next Christendom: The Coming of Global Christianity by Philip Jenkins

The Lost History of Christianity: The Thousand-Year Golden Age of the Church in the Middle East, Africa, and Asia—and How It Died by Philip Jenkins

http://www.answering-islam.org

www.politicalislam.com—Bill Warner's Thirteen Lessons on Political Islam can be downloaded from here.

http://www.cspipublishing.com—All of Bill Warner's books can be ordered here. They include:

An Abridged Koran: the Reconstructed Historical Koran Bill Warner, ed.

A Two Hour Koran Bill Warner, ed.

The Hadith Bill Warner, ed.

The Life of Mohammed Bill Warner, ed.

The following books by Sam Solomon and E. Almaqdisi can be ordered from the ANM website: www.adnamis.org

The Mosque Exposed by Sam Solomon & E. Almaqdisi

The Common Word: the Undermining of the Church by Sam Solomon & E. Almaqdisi

Modern Day Trojan Horse: the Islamic Doctrine of Immigration by Sam Solomon & E. Almaqdisi

Al-Yahud: Eternal Islamic Enmity and the Jews by E. Almaqdisi & Sam Solomon

CPSIA information can be obtained at www.ICGtesting.com
Printed in the USA
BVOW07s0752210114

342540BV00002B/8/P